The International Code of
Marketing of Breast-milk Substitutes

A Common Review
and Evaluation
Framework

WHO/NUT/ 96 2
Distribution General
Original English

The International Code of
Marketing of Breast-milk Substitutes

A Common Review and Evaluation Framework

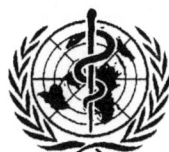

Nutrition Unit
Division of Food and Nutrition
World Health Organization
Geneva
1997

Preface

The Thirty-fourth World Health Assembly (May 1981) adopted the International Code of Marketing of Breast-milk Substitutes in the form of a recommendation and urged all Member States *inter alia* to translate it into national legislation, regulations or other suitable measures; to involve all concerned parties in its implementation; and to monitor compliance with it. The Assembly requested the Director-General of WHO to give all possible support to Member States for the Code's implementation.

During the period 1990–1991, with funds provided by the Government of the Netherlands, and in collaboration with the Government of Sweden and the Swedish International Development Authority, WHO provided technical support to 14 Member States that had indicated a desire to undertake an in-depth review and evaluation of their own experiences in giving effect to the Code. Governments used for this purpose a common review and evaluation framework (CREF) prepared by WHO.

The original CREF has been revised and expanded in the light of the experience gained in using it by the 14 Member States whose representatives met in The Hague in 1991, and the lessons of Member States generally in giving effect to the principles and aim of the Code since its adoption. The revised CREF was also field-tested in Ecuador and Thailand in 1995 and further refined in the light of experience.

The competent authorities and all other concerned parties in countries are invited to use the CREF as a standardized method of information and data collection, adapting it where appropriate, to review and evaluate relevant national action and to monitor progress over time.

Contents

Preface .... *i*

Contents .... *iii*

Glossary of terms .... *vi*

Acknowledgements .... *vii*

Introduction *1*

Structure *4*

Suggested methodologies *6*

Preamble and articles of the International Code *8*

Article 1	Aim of the Code	10
Article 2	Scope of the Code	11
Article 3	Definitions	13
Article 4	Information and education	15
Article 5	The general public and mothers	18
Article 6	Health care systems	20
Article 7	Health workers	23
Article 8	Persons employed by manufacturers and distributors	25
Article 9	Labelling	26
Article 10	Quality	27
Article 11	Implementation and monitoring	29

Conclusion *32*

Annexes

Supporting documentation *33*

Annex 1
The International Code of Marketing of Breast-milk Substitutes 35

Annex 2
Resolutions of the World Health Assembly with particular
reference to the International Code of Marketing of
Breast-milk Substitutes 47

Annex 3
In-depth review and evaluation of national action taken to give effect
to the International Code of Marketing of Breast-milk Substitutes: recommendations
of a technical meeting 53

Suggested frameworks *59*

Annex 4
Suggested framework for assessing informational and educational
materials intended to reach mothers and the general public 61

Annex 5
Suggested framework for assessing informational materials about infant
formula provided to, or for the use of, health professionals 65

Annex 6
Suggested framework for assessing the adequacy of labels
on products within the scope of the Code 67

Annex 7
Suggested framework for conducting site visits 73

Sample questionnaires... *75*

Annex 8

1. Sample questionnaire for the competent national
   authorities (government leaders in health, social welfare
   and related sectors) 77
2. Sample questionnaire for professional associations,
   nongovernmental organizations, and consumer and mother-
   support groups 85
3. Sample questionnaire for mothers in hospital maternity
   wards 93
4. Sample questionnaire for directors of nursing, medical
   directors, and administrators in maternity hospitals, wards
   and clinics 99
5. Sample questionnaire for health facility purchasing
   officers 107
6. Sample questionnaire for health professionals working in
   maternity hospitals, wards and clinics 111
7. Sample questionnaire for community-based health
   professionals 119
8. Sample questionnaire for retailers and retail
   pharmacists 127

Glossary of terms

The thirteen terms explicitly defined in Article 3 of the International Code (Annex 1) have the same meaning in the present context. In addition, the following eight terms are used in the present document as described below.

The principles and aim of the International Code of Marketing of Breast-milk Substitutes means all essential elements laid down in the Code's preamble and articles.

Competent authorities means governments of Member States, or the persons, institutions or organizations that governments have designated as being responsible for the health, nutrition and related social welfare needs of infants and young children and, in particular, for giving effect to the principles and aim of the International Code.

National action/national measures means whatever legislative, administrative or other steps the competent authorities have taken to give effect to the International Code.

CREF means a Common Review and Evaluation Framework, which the competent authorities in Member States are invited to use, adapting it where appropriate, to review and evaluate national action taken to give effect to the International Code.

Assessment team means those persons who have been designated by the competent authorities as being responsible, whether on a permanent or ad hoc basis, for reviewing and evaluating the impact of national action taken to give effect to the International Code.

Key informants means the main individuals in the health and related sectors from whom the assessment team will seek information during the course of reviewing and evaluating national action taken to give effect to the International Code.

Products within the scope of the Code, or national action or measures means those products that are included in the Code's Article 2. They also include any other products that the competent authorities have decided should be specifically included within the scope of national action.

All concerned parties means governments; health authorities, health care systems and the health professionals and other workers employed in them; appropriate nongovernmental, including women's and consumer, organizations, professional groups, institutions, and individuals; and manufacturers and distributors of products within the scope of the International Code.

Acknowledgements

For their unique contribution to the present document, special thanks are due to:

- The Government of the Netherlands for its long-term interest in, and financial support for, the development and application of the CREF, in collaboration with the Government of Sweden and the Swedish International Development Authority.

- The Governments of Australia, Brazil, Egypt, Finland, Guatemala, Islamic Republic of Iran, Kenya, Netherlands, Nigeria, Papua New Guinea, Philippines, Poland, Sweden, United Kingdom of Great Britain and Northern Ireland, and Yemen for applying the first version of the CREF and providing valuable feedback to WHO on their experience (Annex 2).

- The Australian Federal Department of Health and Human Services for providing models that served as the basis for some of the sample questionnaires (Annex 8) in the revised CREF.

- The Governments of Ecuador and Thailand for their willingness to field-test the draft revised CREF.

- The Institute for Reproductive Health, Georgetown University Medical Center, Washington DC—a WHO collaborating centre—for participating in the preparation of the original CREF.

- Rosalind Escott, International Board Certified Lactation Consultant (IBCLC) and community member of the Advisory Panel for the Marketing in Australia of Infant Formula, who was instrumental in preparing the draft revised CREF and collaborated directly in its field-testing in Thailand.

- The numerous international agencies, WHO collaborating centres, nongovernmental organizations and individuals who generously provided comments on the draft revised CREF.

Introduction

In 1979, WHO and UNICEF convened a landmark meeting on infant and young child feeding (1) with representatives of governments, agencies of the United Nations system, nongovernmental organizations, the infant-food industry, and experts in related disciplines. Discussions were organized around five themes:

- The encouragement and support of breast-feeding.
- The promotion and support of appropriate and timely complementary feeding with the use of local food resources.
- The strengthening of education, training and information on infant and young child feeding.
- The development of support for improved health and social status of women in relation to infant and young child health and feeding.
- The appropriate marketing and distribution of breast-milk substitutes.

Following discussions, a statement on infant and young child feeding and a series of recommendations were prepared and adopted by consensus (2). The Thirty-third World Health Assembly (1980), in resolution WHA33.32 (3), subsequently endorsed the statement and recommendations in their entirety; made particular mention of the recommendation that "there should be an international code of marketing of infant formula and other products used as breast-milk substitutes"; and requested the Director-General to prepare such a code "in close consultation with Member States and all other parties concerned including such scientific and other experts whose collaboration may be deemed appropriate".

On 21 May 1981, the Thirty-fourth World Health Assembly adopted the International Code of Marketing of Breast-milk Substitutes (4) (**Annex 1**) in the form of a recommendation and urged all Member States *inter alia* to translate it into national legislation, regulations or other suitable measures; to involve all concerned parties in its implementation; and to monitor compliance with it.

Resolution WHA34.22 by which the Health Assembly adopted the Code stressed that adherence to it "is a minimum requirement and only one of several important actions required in order to protect healthy practices in respect of infant and young child feeding". The implication is that governments, acting individually, are not only permitted to adopt additional, possibly more stringent, measures than those set out in the Code; they are, in effect, actively encouraged to do so. While the Code is not a legally binding instrument as such, it nevertheless represents an expression of the collective will of the membership of the World Health Organization, which has been formally subscribed to by a large number of its Member States, international and regional bodies, nongovernmental organizations and others.

In pursuance of its aim (Article 1), the International Code sets out detailed provisions with regard to:

- Products within its scope (Article 2), in keeping with definitions formulated for the purposes of the Code (Article 3).
- The appropriate dissemination of information and education on infant feeding (Article 4).
- Advertising or other forms of promotion to the general public of products within the scope of the Code (Article 5).
- Measures to be taken in health care systems, and with regard to health workers and employees of manufacturers and distributors (Articles 6, 7 and 8).
- The labelling and quality of breast-milk substitutes and related products (Articles 9 and 10).
- The Code's implementation and monitoring (Article 11).

Where the last is concerned, the Code provides for annual reporting by Member States to the Director-General (Article 11.6) and by the Director-General to the Health Assembly in even years on the status of its implementation (Article 11.7).

Since 1981, the Health Assembly has adopted a number of resolutions dealing *inter alia* with the International Code (see below, for example, in connection with Article 6). While these resolutions do not formally amend the Code, they nevertheless convey the collective views of WHO Member States on the subject. Thus, when Member States seek to develop policies in this area, they may well choose to refer not only to the Code itself but also to subsequent relevant Assembly resolutions (see *inter alia* **Annex 2**).

In May 1990 the Forty-third World Health Assembly requested the Director-General "to support Member States ... in adopting measures to improve infant and young child nutrition, *inter alia* by collecting and disseminating information on relevant action of interest to all Member States" (resolution WHA43.3) (5).

With funds provided by the Government of the Netherlands, and in collaboration with the Government of Sweden and the Swedish International Development Authority, WHO provided technical support to 14 Member States that had indicated a desire to undertake an in-depth review and evaluation of their own experiences in giving effect to the International Code. Governments used for this purpose a common review and evaluation framework (CREF) prepared by WHO.

The original CREF has been revised and expanded in the light of the experience gained in using it by the 14 Member States whose representatives met in The Hague in 1991 (**Annex 3**), and the lessons of Member States generally in giving effect to the principles and aim of the International Code since 1981. Indeed, reports by the Director-General to the World Health Assembly in even years between 1982 and 1996 provide a detailed account, totalling more than 300 pages, of the steps taken by 161 countries and territories—individually, and in some cases collectively, through regional and interregional forums—to give effect to the Code (6). The revised CREF was field-tested in Ecuador and Thailand in 1995 and further refined in the light of experience.

To the extent that resources permit, WHO stands ready to give Member States all possible support, as and when requested, for implementing the International Code and, in particular, in preparing national legislation, regulations or other suitable measures, as well as in applying the CREF to review and evaluate national action (7).

References

1. Joint WHO/UNICEF Meeting on Infant and Young Child Feeding, Geneva, 9-12 October 1979.

2. Document WHA33/1980/REC/1, Annex 6.

3. Handbook of resolutions and decisions, Vol. II, 1985, pp. 90-91.

4. World Health Organization. *International Code of Marketing of Breast-milk Substitutes*. Document WHA34/1981/REC/1, Annex 3, Geneva, 1981.

5. Resolution WHA43.3 (*Handbook of resolutions and decisions of the World Health Assembly and the Executive Board*, Volume III, 3rd ed., Geneva, 1993, p. 64).

6. Relevant information from progress reports between 1982 and 1990 has been combined into a single document (WHO/MCH/NUT/90.1). Complementing this synthesis is a second document (WHO/HLE/NUT/92.1) that focuses on the Code's individual articles and describes how each has been given expression through national legislation and other suitable measures. Progress reports presented to the Health Assembly in even years from 1982 to 1994 are found in annex to the corresponding volume 1 of WHO official records.

7. With regard to sources for national authorities of information and documentation on measures that have been adopted in various countries to give effect to the International Code, see the recommendations of the technical meeting in The Hague (Annex 3) under the heading "development and implementation".

Structure

The competent authorities and all other concerned parties in countries are invited to use the CREF, adapting it where appropriate, to review and evaluate relevant national action. The CREF covers the preamble and articles of the International Code, and each section is divided into three parts:

A summary box which describes the main focus of the preamble and each article.

Issues which includes a number of primary and secondary topics that could serve to define the situation with respect to the preamble and each article.

Key informants which suggests where information may be found concerning those questions of greatest relevance to implementing national infant feeding policy, including the International Code.

The CREF has been designed to facilitate review and evaluation of national action by focusing on collection and analysis of information that will permit the assessment team to:

- Describe what action has been taken, or is under way, to give effect to the International Code, in whole or in part.
- Identify factors that have facilitated or hindered action.
- Assess the impact of action on the basis of locally suitable indicators.
- Make appropriate recommendations.

The CREF follows the order established in the Code, referring, where appropriate, to relevant resolutions of the World Health Assembly. However, because the preamble and articles are all closely interrelated, the Code should be viewed as a whole. In analysing each provision, the assessment team may wish to:

- Describe the legislation, regulations, policies, standards of practice, agreements, administrative decisions, or other relevant measures that have been adopted, or are in the process of being adopted, to give effect to the principles and aim of the International Code, including details of relevant sanctions applied.

- Record, e.g. through interviews and surveys, the perceptions of policy-makers, programme managers, health service providers, mothers and other child care-givers, and other concerned parties about the nature and impact of national action taken to give effect to the Code.
- Learn how national action is being implemented among the general public and manufacturers and distributors, and within the health care system.
- Determine, e.g. through focus-group interviews and observations, whether there have been any changes in the perceptions and practices of mothers as a result of national action to give effect to the Code.
- Observe the nature and origin of difficulties encountered in the process of giving effect to the Code and efforts being made to overcome them.

As noted above, **Annex 1** reproduces the International Code in its entirety while **Annex 2** reproduces two resolutions of the World Health Assembly with particular reference to the International Code. **Annex 3** contains the recommendations of a technical meeting based on some Member States' experience with implementing the Code. **Annex 4** provides a suggested framework to assess informational and educational materials (Article 4) intended to reach mothers and the general public; **Annex 5** is a suggested framework for assessing informational materials provided by manufacturers and distributors to health professionals regarding products within the scope of the Code (Article 7); and **Annex 6** is a suggested framework for assessing adequacy of product labels (Article 9). Finally, **Annex 7** provides a list of observations that the assessment team could use to structure site visits to health care facilities (Article 6) and **Annex 8** a series of sample questionnaires that could be used to obtain relevant information from key informants.

Suggested methodologies

The assessment team may wish to avail itself of some or all of the following methodologies.

Literature and data desk review

Prior to conducting any field activity, the assessment team would no doubt find it useful to gather all relevant background information. This material can be reviewed for content and context in documenting pre-existing behaviour. It can also be used as a basis for preparing a chronological review of national action taken to give effect to the International Code.

Key informant interviews and surveys

The assessment team can draw up a list of key informants, including the competent authorities, professional associations, nongovernmental organizations, consumer and mother-support groups, health professionals in administrative and clinical positions, and manufacturers, distributors and retailers of products within the scope of the Code and national measures to give effect to it. Key informants could be interviewed using questionaries developed for this purpose (**Annex 8**). The information thus obtained should assist in answering the questions in each of the "issues" sections of each article of the Code.

The assessment team can use questionnaires as a basis for conducting both interviews and wider surveys. Information should be collected so as to describe both the perceptions of the individuals interviewed with respect to actual practices within the health care system and to provide an objective means of documenting what is actually occurring. Responses will enable the team to identify where additional information may be required. A principal criterion for selecting priority issues for closer examination could be their impact on successful implementation of national policy to protect, promote and support breast-feeding.

Site visits

Site visits by the assessment team could include observations and interviews with key informants (**Annex 7**). The team may also wish to interview small groups of health workers, health facility administrators, pharmacists and other retail traders, and mothers of breast-fed and non-breast-fed infants (**Annex 8**, sample questionnaires 2 and 3) . If the expertise is available, these interviews could follow standard focus-group approaches. However, group interviews exploring the same questions will in any case yield valuable information. In addition, if information about infant feeding patterns is available, it could be compared to other data sources as appropriate.

Review of relevant protocols, texts, information materials, and record forms

Through site visits, interviews, surveys and other contacts, the assessment team could collect, and review for accuracy and appropriateness, all relevant printed materials, e.g. the breast-feeding content of delivery-room protocols and infant health reviews. Relevant forms can be obtained directly from health care facilities (**Annex 8**, sample questionnaires 4, 5 and 6). Of particular importance in this context are the practices in maternity wards and hospitals that have been designated "baby-friendly" in accordance with the principles laid down in the joint WHO/UNICEF statement on breast-feeding and maternity services (1).

Historical review of the print media

Where possible, a historical review of popular magazines and professional journals, or other regularly distributed materials for mothers and health professionals, should be carried out. Examples can be reviewed for the number of articles on infant-feeding topics and their context, and for specific advertisements and their content.

Reference

1. In 1991 WHO and the United Nations Children's Fund (UNICEF) jointly launched the Baby-friendly Hospital Initiative, which aims to give every baby the best start in life by ensuring a health care environment where breast-feeding is the norm. The initiative is based on the principals summarized in *Protecting, promoting and supporting breast-feeding: the special role of maternity services*. A joint WHO/ UNICEF statement (Geneva, World Health Organization, 1989). By 1996, this statement had been translated into more than 40 languages and more than 8000 hospitals had been selected to achieve "baby-friendly" status in 171 countries.

Preamble and articles of the International Code

Preamble

The preamble to the International Code generally summarizes the Code's main underlying principles, including why usual marketing practices are unsuitable for breast-milk substitutes. It emphasises that breast-feeding is an unequalled way of providing food for the healthy growth and development of infants; that it forms a unique biological and emotional basis for the health of both mothers and children; and that the anti-infective properties of breast milk help to protect infants against disease. The preamble acknowledges that "when mothers do not breast-feed, or only do so partially, there is a legitimate market for infant formula". Infant formula and suitable ingredients from which to prepare it should accordingly be made accessible to those who need them. However, they should not be marketed or distributed in ways that may interfere with the protection and promotion of breast-feeding. The preamble also stresses the importance of breast-feeding for infants, their vulnerability in the early months of life, and the risks associated with inappropriate feeding practices, while drawing attention to the impact that improper practices in the marketing of breast-milk substitutes and related products can have on infant malnutrition, morbidity and mortality in all countries. The preamble stresses the essential role of governments, heath care systems, health workers, educational systems, social services, communities, and nongovernmental organizations in protecting and promoting breast-feeding; it also recalls that manufacturers and distributors of breast-milk substitutes have an important and constructive role to play both in relation to infant feeding and in promoting the aim of the Code and its proper implementation. The preamble states that governments should undertake a variety of measures to promote healthy growth and development of infants and young children, and notes that the Code concerns only one aspect of these measures. Finally, governments are called upon to take action appropriate to their social and legislative framework to give effect to the principles and aim of the Code, including the enactment of legislation, regulations or other suitable measures.

Issues

0.1 The degree of commitment by the competent authorities to implementing the Code in its entirety.

0.2 The degree of commitment, by all other parties concerned, to full implementation of the Code.

0.3 The extent to which all parties concerned understand why breast-feeding is important and why the marketing of breast-milk substitutes requires special treatment.

0.4 Other measures to protect and promote breast-feeding that have been taken, or are in effect, involving the health care system (e.g. implementation of the Baby-friendly Hospital Initiative), health workers, the educational system, social services, communities and mother-support and other organizations.

Key informants

- Policy-makers.
- Senior health and nutrition authorities at national and regional levels.
- Heads of nongovernmental organizations and professional societies.

See **Annex 8**, sample questionnaires 1 and 2.

Article 1
Aim of the Code

Article 1 describes the aim of the Code and places it in the context of infants' broader health and nutritional needs. Achieving the aim—contributing to the provision of safe and adequate nutrition for infants—means protecting and promoting breast-feeding, and ensuring the proper use of breast-milk substitutes, when they are necessary, on the basis of adequate information and through appropriate marketing and distribution.

Issues

1.1 Is achieving the aim of the Code adequately reflected in national health policy and practice?

1.2 What is the status of national action taken to give effect to the Code? For example, has explicit national or state/provincial legislation or other suitable measures been adopted corresponding to all, or most, of the articles of the International Code?

1.3 Has national action been taken by enacting new, or broadening existing, regulations, directives, agreements, or guidelines? Has such action included all the Code's articles?

1.4 Has action also been effected through administrative, voluntary or other means?

1.5 Is there any legislation that limits or enhances achievement of the Code's aim?

Key informants

- Policy-makers, senior health and nutrition authorities at national and regional levels, legal authorities responsible for health and marketing legislation and regulations, nongovernmental organizations and professional societies.

See **Annex 8**, sample questionnaires 1 and 2.

Article 2
Scope of the Code

Article 2 describes the food products that are covered by the International Code, including their quality and availability and information concerning their use, and feeding bottles and teats. Food products other than *bona fide* breast-milk substitutes, including infant formula—e.g. other milk products, foods and beverages, including bottle-fed complementary foods—are covered by the Code only when they are "marketed or otherwise represented to be suitable ... for use as a partial or total replacement of breast milk" (1). However, taking into account both the intent and the spirit of the International Code, WHO has observed (2) that there would appear to be grounds for the competent authorities in countries to decide that a product or products, e.g. follow-up formula, fall within the scope of the International Code in the light of the way the product or products are used in individual circumstances. Perception and use could serve as a measure of the impact of the phrase "otherwise represented to be suitable" in the Code's Article 2.

Issues

2.1 Have national measures been adopted to give effect to the International Code? If so, do they cover all products within the scope of the Code?

2.2 Is the scope of national action identical to, or broader or narrower than, the Code (3)?

2.3 Are products other than *bona fide* breast-milk substitutes, including infant formula, being marketed or otherwise represented to be suitable for use as a partial or total replacement of breast milk?

2.4 Of the products that are marketed for infant feeding, are any commonly *used* as a replacement for breast milk, even if they are not formally marketed as such?

2.5 Are any products being marketed or used for infant feeding that do not fall within the scope of national action?

2.6　Does national action cover the quality and availability of all products within the scope of the Code?

2.7　Does national action include specifications for the form and content of information concerning the use of all products within the scope of the Code?

Resource documents and materials

- Copies of legislation, regulations, directives and agreements, and a detailed comparison of each text relative to the International Code.

- Examples of promotional materials used in marketing products for infant feeding.

See **Annex 8**, sample questionnaire 1.

References

1. See excerpts from the Introductory Statement by the Representative of the Executive Board to the Thirty-fourth World Health Assembly on the subject of the Draft International Code of Marketing of Breast-milk Substitutes. Document WHA34/1981/REC/3, page 188.

2. Infant and young child nutrition (progress and evaluation report; and status of the International Code of Marketing of Breast-milk Substitutes). Report by the Director-General to the Forty-fifth World Health Assembly, document WHA45/1992/REC/1, Annex 9, paragraph 49.

3. Participants in the 1991 technical meeting in The Hague on the review and evaluation of national action (see Annex 3) considered that difficulties encountered in developing and implementing national measures to give effect to the International Code included "questions relating to the scope of the Code, including (a) products that are sometimes erroneously perceived and used as breast-milk substitutes, e.g. starchy gruels, herbal teas and follow-up formula; (b) the absence of internationally recognized quality and design standards for feeding bottles and teats; and (c) problems related to other infant-feeding utensils, e.g. feeding cups with perforated lips, and dummies" (document WHO/MCH/NUT/91.2, paragraph 8).

Article 3
Definitions

Article 3 is straightforward at first glance, defining precisely the meaning of the terms used in the specific context of the International Code. National legislation, regulations and other measures frequently use identical or very similar definitions. However, these definitions are occasionally applied in ways that are inconsistent with the original, for example a blurring of the distinction between "samples" of products within the scope of the Code, which are generally prohibited, and donations or low-priced sales of "supplies", which are permitted only under certain very limited conditions (see Article 6).

Issues

3.1   Which of the terms defined in this article are included in national action taken to give effect to the International Code?

3.2   Are the Code's original definitions used? Do alternative definitions strengthen or weaken achievement of the Code's principles and aim?

3.3   Have additional terms been defined for purposes of national action?

Key informants

- Policy-makers.
- Senior health and nutrition authorities.
- Legal authorities responsible for health and marketing legislation and regulations.
- Staff of academic or research institutions who may be asked to provide technical guidance.
- Heads of professional societies and nongovernmental organizations.

Every effort should be made to distinguish between definitions used in national action and the understanding of those persons responsible for applying them.

Resource documents

- Copies of legislation, regulations, directives, guidelines, agreements, and descriptions of action taken compared with the International Code. Check copies held at various levels and in different institutions to see whether any inconsistencies appear or whether the texts have been adapted differently in different settings.

See **Annex 8,** sample questionnaire 1.

Article 4
Information and education

A key element here is the objectivity and consistency of information, but equally important is the responsibility of the competent authorities for its provision, planning, design, and dissemination, or their control. Article 4 covers informational and educational materials such as pamphlets, booklets and audiovisual materials intended to reach families and those involved in the field of infant and young child nutrition. This article thus covers client/consumer/patient education texts and other instructional materials in a variety of formats, including audio, video and print. Materials covered by this article are required to include information on specified points. There are a number of restrictions on the distribution and content of materials donated by manufacturers or distributors.

Issues

4.1   Do the competent authorities take responsibility for the information provided to families?

4.2   How do the competent authorities carry out this responsibility, directly or indirectly, e.g. through nongovernmental or other groups?

4.3   To what extent are the competent authorities involved in the planning, provision, design and dissemination of information?

4.4   Describe the process by which materials are produced for family education and the organizations or bodies responsible for preparing these materials.

4.5   What mechanisms do the competent authorities use to review educational materials or otherwise exercise control over their content to ensure that they contain all the information specified in Article 4.2?

4.6   Do the competent authorities also take responsibility for the information about breast-feeding and infant nutrition that health care providers receive during basic and in-service training?

If yes, please describe how this responsibility is carried out.

If no, describe what authority controls the content of these education programmes.

4.7 Do the competent authorities have a policy governing donations of informational or educational equipment or materials for use by families and/ or in educating health workers?

If yes, please describe the policy and assess its impact, e.g. are donations made at the request of, and with written approval from, the competent authorities or within guidelines governing these donations?

If donations are made, do materials bear the name of any product within the scope of the Code, or any information other than the company's name or logo?

4.8 Is distribution of materials restricted to the health care system?

N.B. In particular, the assessment team should collect and evaluate breast-feeding promotion materials to ensure that they do not undermine breast-feeding by giving incomplete or inaccurate advice, making breast-feeding appear difficult or unattractive, creating doubt in women's minds about their ability to breast-feed, or implying or creating a belief that bottle-feeding is equivalent or superior to breast-feeding.

Key informants

- National legal authorities, and those persons responsible for health education and the production and monitoring of related materials.
- Professional and educational bodies responsible for health care education.
- Directors and administrators of health care facilities.
- Health workers in maternal and child health and nutrition-related services, lactation consultants.
- Mothers, including those attending different types of services.
- Members of breast-feeding support groups.

Resource documents and materials

- Government policy documents, including those possibly delegating authority, concerning informational and educational materials for families and those involved in infant and young child feeding.
- Policies of relevant agencies or organizations.
- Information from other sources, e.g. professional societies or infant-food manufacturers that produce and distribute educational materials.
- Educational materials for families and health care providers.

N.B.   The educational materials collected should be evaluated to see whether they meet the standards laid down in Article 4.2 of the Code or relevant national standards. If possible, interpretation of the materials gathered should be discussed with mothers and their families.

See also **Annex 4** and **Annex 5**.

Article 5
The general public and mothers

Article 5 is a central provision, covering marketing, retailing, advertising, and other forms of promotion to the general public and mothers of products within the scope of the Code. There should be no advertising or other form of promotion of these products, nor should manufacturers and distributors provide, directly or indirectly, samples of products, or gifts which may promote their use.

Issues

5.1   How do national measures deal with advertising, sales inducements, gifts, and product sampling to the general public?

5.2   Describe how national measures might differ from the International Code in the context of Article 5. If they do, state why.

5.3   Do other instruments, such as commercial or trade laws or regulations, codes of practice from professional societies, agreements entered into, or guidelines developed by, manufacturers and distributors affect the marketing of products to the general public?

5.4   If yes, describe the instruments and discuss their history.

5.5   Compare and contrast national policy with actual marketing practices, e.g. has advertising or other form of promotion of products within the scope of the Code ceased, or does it continue despite the adoption of national measures?

5.6   Is there advertising or other promotion to the general public of products that are, strictly speaking, **outside** the scope of the International Code but that is nevertheless incompatible with the principles and aim of the Code, e.g. publicity for mineral water, children's toys, and microwave ovens directly featuring infant formula and feeding bottles and teats?

5.7 Discuss the impact of measures to restrict marketing to the general public of products within the scope of the Code and discuss how practices may have changed over time.

5.8 Discuss with representatives of commercial interests their perspective on the International Code and the regulation of related business practices, and how they describe their adherence to the principles and aim of the Code and national measures adopted to give effect to it.

N.B. Some questions relevant to Article 5 lend themselves to the undertaking of quick surveys. The assessment team can decide whether to conduct studies in conjunction with other means at their disposal for evaluating the impact of marketing to the general public and mothers. If such studies are done, they should follow generally accepted survey methods, especially with respect to choice of sampling frames and use of other quantitative techniques.

Key informants

- Policy-makers.
- Senior health and nutrition authorities at national and regional levels.
- Legal authorities familiar with health and marketing legislation and regulations.
- Nongovernmental organizations and professional societies.
- Responsible media authorities.
- Representatives of the infant-food and feeding-utensil industries; breast-feeding support groups and other nongovernmental organizations.
- Members of the general public.

See **Annex 8**, sample questionnaires 1 to 8.

Article 6
Health care systems

Health care facilities have long been recognized as an attractive venue for promoting, directly or indirectly, infant formula and other products within the scope of the Code (Article 2). Article 6 recognizes this potential for abuse and reminds health authorities that they should "give appropriate information and advice to health workers in regard to their responsibilities" for encouraging and protecting breast-feeding and promoting the Code's principles (6.1).

- The article makes clear (6.2–6.4) that no facility of a health care system should be used for the purpose of promoting products within the scope of the Code, and that no personnel provided or paid for by manufacturers or distributors may be used there. Feeding with infant formula may be demonstrated (6.5), but only by designated persons and only to those who need to use it. Health professionals may receive product information (6.2), but it should be limited to scientific and factual matters, as provided in Article 7.2.

- The article describes (6.6–6.7) the narrow, indeed stringent, circumstances in which "donations or low-price sales ... of supplies of infant formula or other products within the scope of [the] Code, whether for use in institutions or distribution outside them, may be made". The article draws on the Code's precise definition (Article 3) of "supplies" ("quantities of a product provided for use over an extended period, free or at a low price, for social purposes, including those provided to families in need"), in contrast to "samples" ("single or small quantities of a product provided without cost"), which the Code generally seeks to eliminate. Thus, to be legitimate, Article 6 insists that supplies satisfy all three of the following criteria:

  - They should only be used or distributed for infants who have to be fed on breast-milk substitutes.
  - They should not be used as a sales inducement.
  - They should be continued for as long as the infants concerned need them.

Two resolutions of the World Health Assembly urge Member States to take even more stringent action in this regard (see Annex 2). In resolution WHA39.28 (1986), the World Health Assembly concluded that only a minority of infants require breast-milk substitutes in maternity wards and hospitals, and that the small amounts in question should be made available through normal procurement channels and not through free or subsidized supplies. In resolution WHA47.5 (1994) the Health Assembly urged Member States "to ensure that there are no donations of free and subsidized supplies ... in any part of the health care system".

For emergency relief operations, resolution WHA47.5 also calls on Member States "to exercise extreme caution when planning, implementing or supporting emergency relief operations, by protecting, promoting and supporting breast-feeding for infants, and ensuring that donated supplies of breast-milk substitutes ... be given only if all" three of the above criteria are met.

Issues

6.1   What measures have the competent authorities adopted to promote the principles and aim of the Code within the health care system, for example fostering adoption of the principles laid down in the joint WHO/UNICEF statement on breast-feeding and maternity services (1), as part of their implementation of the Baby-friendly Hospital Initiative.

6.2   What role have the competent authorities decided the health care system should play in protecting, promoting and supporting breast-feeding?

6.3   Have the competent authorities taken appropriate measures to educate health workers concerning their responsibilities for encouraging and protecting breast-feeding and promoting the principles of the Code?

6.4   Do health care facilities display, promote, or provide samples (single or small quantities) of products within the scope of the code?

6.5   Do health care facilities encourage the use of products within the scope of the Code?

6.6   Are mothers provided through the health care system printed materials that promote the use of any products within the scope of the Code?

6.7   Do health care facilities distribute material provided by manufacturers and distributors which does not comply with all the conditions specified in Article 4.3?

6.8   Are personnel used in any part of the health care system provided, or paid for, by manufacturers or distributors of products within the scope of the Code?

6.9   Is the correct preparation and feeding of infant formula, including an explanation of the potential health hazards of improper use, demonstrated **only** to mothers or family members who need to use it and **only** by health workers or other community workers as appropriate?

6.10 Do manufacturers or distributors of products within the scope of the Code donate equipment or materials to the health care system?

      If so, do they bear more than a company's name or logo? Is there any mention of, or reference to, products within the scope of the Code?

6.11 Do national measures permit donations or low-price sales of products within the scope of the Code, and, if so, is there a monitoring mechanism for this purpose?

6.12 Which institutions or organizations, if any, are permitted to receive supplies of products within the scope of the Code?

6.13 Is there a difference in the pattern of donations or low-price sales of products within the scope of the Code in different parts of the health care system or between the "public" and the "private" sectors?

6.14 How do the competent authorities provide for the safe and adequate nutrition of socially disadvantaged infants who are not breast-fed? Is this done in a way that does not compromise breast-feeding of other infants?

6.15 Are any so-called "supplies" of products within the scope of the Code, which are provided free or at low cost, in fact being used or distributed as de facto "samples", i.e. small quantities of a product given to many mothers or used in feeding many infants, each for a short period?

Key informants

- Government officials in health, social welfare and other relevant fields.
- Medical and nursing directors and administrators in health facilities.
- Health workers in maternal and child health and nutrition-related services.
- Health workers in private practice.
- Nongovernmental organizations, including consumer and mother-support groups.
- Manufacturers and distributors of products within the scope of the Code.
- Groups or individuals responsible for monitoring application of national measures.
- Administrators in social welfare institutions and organizations
- Social workers.
- Mothers, including those benefiting from various health and social services.

See **Annex 8**, sample questionnaires 1 to 8.

Reference

1. *Protecting, promoting and supporting breast-feeding: the special role of maternity services, op. cit.*

Article 7
Health workers

Article 7 describes health workers' responsibilities under the Code for encouraging and protecting breast-feeding. It also deals with restrictions on the information that manufacturers and distributors may provide health professionals regarding products within the scope of the Code; financial and material inducements from commercial interests, which are not permitted; and contributions to health workers towards educational or research activities, which should be disclosed by both parties. The article contains the only exception to the Code's "no samples" provision—i.e. for the purpose of professional evaluation or research at the institutional level—and reiterates the principle laid down in Article 5.2 that samples of infant formula should not be given to mothers of infants and young children, or to members of health workers' families.

Issues

7.1   Do national measures adopted to give effect to the International Code emphasize health workers' responsibility to protect, promote and support breast-feeding?

7.2   Do national measures include restrictions on the type and scope of information that manufacturers and distributors can provide health workers?

7.3   Do national measures include restrictions on financial and material inducements to health workers from manufacturers and distributors?

7.4   Is there a mechanism to ensure that all contributions by manufacturers and distributors towards educational or research activities for health workers are disclosed by both parties?

7.5   Do national measures ensure that samples of infant formula and other products within the scope of the Code are not provided to health workers except under the stringent conditions specified in this article?

7.6 Have steps been taken to ensure that samples of infant formula and other products within the scope of the Code are not given to mothers or members of their families?

7.7 Do the competent authorities formally assess the scientific and factual content of information provided by manufacturers and distributors regarding products within the scope of the Code?

N.B. It is suggested that all such materials be collected and analysed using a standardized assessment tool.

Key informants

- This article can most easily be evaluated by interviewing members of the various professions working in health facilities, and by collecting product-related printed and audiovisual materials used by health workers. The assessment team can decide how many, and which categories, of health workers should be interviewed and where, although a range of personnel is desirable. An efficient way to do this would be to seek out different categories of health workers, including paediatricians, obstetricians/gynaecologists, nurses, midwives, nutritionists, dietitians, and lactation consultants, at meetings of their professional associations.

Information materials

- The assessment team should request the different categories of health workers to provide examples of pamphlets, posters, product information, and so forth that they receive from manufacturers and distributors of products within the scope of the Code. These materials should be examined to see whether they comply with the Code's Articles 4 and 7.

See **Annex 4** and **Annex 5**.

Article 8
Persons employed by manufacturers and distributors

Article 8 restricts sales incentives for marketing personnel, but only for products within the scope of the Code. There should be no sales quotas, or links between bonuses and the volume of sales. Marketing personnel are also restricted from performing educational functions for mothers or the general public. However, written approval from the competent authorities may be given for them to be used for other functions within the health care system.

Issues

8.1 Do national measures prohibit sales incentives for marketing personnel linked to the volume of sales of products within the scope of the Code?

8.2 Do manufacturers and distributors set quotas for marketing personnel, bonuses or other sales incentives for products within the scope of the Code?

8.3 Do persons employed by manufacturers of distributors of products within the scope of the Code perform any educational functions within the health care system? If so, on whose behalf? Who is this authorized by?

8.4 Are marketing personnel authorized to perform other functions within the health care system? What are these functions and are there any restrictions in this regard?

Key informants

- In addition to persons employed by manufacturers and distributors, the assessment team may wish to confirm responses received through interviews with health care programme managers, health care providers, and representatives of nongovernmental organizations.

See **Annex 8**, sample questionnaires 1 to 8.

Article 9
Labelling

Article 9 describes the required balance between providing necessary information about products within the scope of the Code and their use while simultaneously avoiding any discouragement of breast-feeding. Specified information should be clearly and conspicuously provided in an appropriate language. Pictures of infants, or any pictures, text or words that may idealize the use of a product, may not be used. Labels should enable easy identification of a product, and give clear instructions on how to prepare and use it. Products suitable for modification for use as a breast-milk substitute should carry a warning that the unmodified product should not be the sole source of nourishment for an infant. The label should also provide information on ingredients, composition/analysis, storage conditions, and batch number and date for use. The article singles out sweetened condensed milk as being totally unsuitable for infant feeding, or for use as a main ingredient for infant formula; its label should thus not contain purported instructions on how to modify it for that purpose.

Issues

The labels of products within the scope of the Code, plus the labels of other products which might be marketed as breast-milk substitutes, should be reviewed under this article. It is suggested that examples of relevant materials be collected, and assessed using a standardized assessment tool.

Documents and materials

- The labels of all products within the scope of the Code, plus the labels of other products which might be marketed as breast-milk substitutes.

See **Annex 6** for a suggested framework for assessing adequacy of labels on products within the scope of the Code.

Article 10
Quality

Article 10 seeks to protect the health of infants by ensuring that products within the scope of the Code comply with high recognized standards. Food products should meet applicable standards and codes of practice recommended by the Codex Alimentarius Commission, which should apply whether the products are manufactured locally or imported. During the technical meeting in The Hague in 1991 (see introduction and Annex 3) concern was expressed over the absence of internationally recognized standards for the quality and design of feeding bottles and teats (nipples).

Issues

10.1 Have the competent authorities accepted the relevant Codex standards (1) or adopted more stringent ones?

10.2 Are the standards being observed by all concerned parties?

10.3 Is there any cause for concern about the quality and/or design of feeding bottles and teats (2) available for sale on the domestic market?

10.4 What methods, e.g. periodic or regular inspection, are used to ensure product quality?

Key informants

• Competent national authorities, including Codex Alimentarius contact points.

Documents and materials

• Relevant Codex standards.
• Relevant national legislation.

See **Annex 8**, sample questionnaire 1.

References

1. The Codex standard for Infant Formula (CODEX STAN 72-1981) and the Recommended Code of Hygienic Practice for Foods for Infants and Children (CAC/RCP 21-1979) are found in Volume 4 of the *Codex Alimentarius*. Rome, Food and Agriculture Organization of the United Nations, 1994.

2. For feeding a breast-milk substitute, WHO recommends the use of a cup, which is easily cleaned. If bottles and teats are used, they should be designed so that they can be thoroughly cleaned and are able to withstand boiling. Participants in the technical meeting on the review and evaluation of national action (The Hague, 1991, see **Annex 3**) expressed the view that "too little attention has been paid to regulating the marketing and promotion of feeding bottles and teats, and other devices including dummies (also known as pacifiers or soothers) and feeding cups with perforated lids. In addition, there are no internationally recognized standards for the quality and design of feeding bottles and teats" (document WHO/MCH/NUT/91.2, paragraph 39).

Article 11
Implementation and monitoring

This provision calls on governments to give effect to the principles and aim of the International Code, as appropriate to their social and legislative framework, and recalls that technical support is available for this purpose if desired. It refers to the responsibility governments have for monitoring the application of the Code, whether acting individually, or collectively through the World Health Organization, and calls on all concerned parties to collaborate with governments to this end. Member States are meant to report annually to the Director-General on action taken, and the Director-General to the Health Assembly, in even years, on the status of the Code's implementation. Manufacturers and distributors of products within the scope of the Code are held responsible for monitoring their marketing practices according to the principles and aim of the Code. Other concerned parties are invited to draw the attention of manufacturers or distributors to activities which are incompatible with the principles and aim of the Code, while ensuring that the appropriate governmental authority is also informed.

Issues

11.1 In keeping with the national social and legislative framework, what specific actions, e.g. adoption of legislation, regulations, directives, policy statements, guidelines, special instructions, administrative circulars, agreements or other suitable measures, have the competent authorities taken to give effect to the principles and aim of the Code?

11.2 Has the cooperation of WHO, UNICEF, or any other agency of the United Nations system been sought in this connection?

11.3 Has relevant national action, including laws and regulations, taken to give effect to the principles and aim of the Code been publicly stated, and does it apply on the same basis to all those involved in the manufacture and marketing of products within its scope?

11.4 Is there a system for monitoring application of national action taken to give effect to the principles and aim of the Code and has responsibility for monitoring been formally assigned (1)?

11.5 If there is a system, does it include regular collection of information, using epidemiological studies or other suitable methods (see **Annex 8**), on the number and scale of violations of national action taken to give effect to the International Code?

11.6 Do manufacturers and distributors, nongovernmental organizations, professional groups, and consumer organizations collaborate with the competent authorities in monitoring application of the Code?

11.7 Do manufacturers and distributors engage in "self-monitoring", i.e. do they monitor their marketing practices according to the principles and aim of the Code, and do they do this independently of any other action taken to implement the Code?

11.8 Do nongovernmental organizations (2), professional groups, and concerned individuals inform the competent authorities of any activities of manufacturers or distributors which are deemed to be incompatible with the principles and aim of the Code?

11.9 If so, what action is taken to correct the situation and what sanctions (3) can be applied?

11.10 Have manufacturers and primary distributors apprised their marketing personnel of the Code and their responsibilities under it?

11.11 Does the competent authority contribute to collective monitoring of the Code, through the World Health Organization, by regularly communicating to the Director-General of WHO information on action taken to give effect to the principles and aim of the Code?

Key informants

- Competent national authorities.
- All other concerned parties.

Documents and materials

- Copies of legal and other relevant instruments or texts adopted to give effect to the principles and aim of the Code, including legislation, regulations, directives, policy statements, guidelines, special instructions, administrative circulars, agreements or other suitable measures.
- Copies of instruments providing for settlement of disputes regarding application of the Code nationally, e.g. by an ombudsman, conciliation group, or monitoring committee.
- Copies of complaints, if any, alleging non-observance of national measures, and their resolution.

See **Annex 8**, sample questionnaires 1 to 8.

References

1. Participants in the technical meeting in The Hague (1991) on the review and evaluation of national action to give effect to the Code (**Annex 3**) observed that "the monitoring of measures adopted to give effect to the International Code, often with the support of national and international nongovernmental organizations, has been successful in some countries. In many other countries, however, monitoring has proved to be absent, poorly planned, or ineffective for lack of the proper designation of responsibilities among those concerned. Other factors contributing to incomplete monitoring are an absence of baseline data, trained staff, appropriate indicators, and adequate funding" (document WHO/MCH/NUT/91.2, paragraph 31).

2. The International Baby Food Action Network (IBFAN, P.O. Box 19, 10700 Penang, Malaysia, Tel. +60 4 656 9799, Fax +60 4 657 7291), with more than 140 member organizations in some 70 countries, periodically holds training courses on implementing the International Code for participants from developing countries. Course content includes the policy, socioeconomic and legal dimensions of the Code, and individual guidance and references are provided. Participants also have access to the extensive range of related materials, including periodic IBFAN surveys of Code implementation, collected by the Code documentation centre on the premises.

3. Participants in the technical meeting on the review and evaluation of national action (The Hague, 1991; see **Annex 3**) observed that "difficulties encountered in enforcing national measures include absence of sanctions, inadequate sanctions or inability to apply them in practices, and provisions that require subjective interpretations on the part of national authorities" (document WHO/MCH/NUT/91.2, paragraph 32).

Conclusion

On completing their review and evaluation exercise, the competent authorities may wish to summarize how far they consider national action to have gone in giving effect to the principles and aim of the Code. Later, the competent authorities, with the help of the assessment team could summarize:

- Action that has been taken, or is in the process of being taken, to give effect to the International Code.
- Factors which have facilitated or hindered action.
- The impact of action taken on the marketing patterns of breast-milk substitutes and breast-feeding prevalence and duration (1).

Having established a baseline by undertaking a thorough review and evaluation of national action to give effect to the International Code, the competent authorities may wish to update their information periodically through interviews and observations at a small number of sites. To ensure the effectiveness of any update, all concerned parties should be given the opportunity to contribute. Particular emphasis should be placed on identifying those areas requiring additional attention in keeping with changes in breast-feeding prevalence and duration and evolving marketing and distribution practices both for products within the scope of the International Code and other products within the scope of relevant national measures.

Reference

1. WHO welcomes information on the prevalence and duration of breast-feeding for inclusion in its global breast-feeding database, which was restructured in 1993-1994 using new indicators. For a complete description see document WHO/NUT/96.1 *Global Data Bank on Breast-feeding*, which is available on request from the Nutrition unit, World Health Organization, 1211 Geneva 27, Switzerland.

Supporting documentation

Annex 1

The International Code of Marketing of Breast-milk Substitutes 35

Annex 2

Resolutions of the World Health Assembly with particular reference
to the International Code of Marketing of Breast-milk Substitutes 47

Annex 3

In-depth review and evaluation of national action taken to give effect
to the International Code of Marketing of Breast-milk Substitutes:
recommendations of a technical meeting 53

International Code of Marketing of Breast-milk Substitutes (1)

The Member States of the World Health Organization:

Affirming the right of every child and every pregnant and lactating woman to be adequately nourished as a means of attaining and maintaining health;

Recognizing that infant malnutrition is part of the wider problems of lack of education, poverty, and social injustice;

Recognizing that the health of infants and young children cannot be isolated from the health and nutrition of women, their socioeconomic status and their roles as mothers;

Conscious that breast-feeding is an unequalled way of providing ideal food for the healthy growth and development of infants; that it forms a unique biological and emotional basis for the health of both mother and child; that the anti-infective properties of breast milk help to protect infants against disease; and that there is an important relationship between breast-feeding and child-spacing;

Recognizing that the encouragement and protection of breast-feeding is an important part of the health, nutrition and other social measures required to promote healthy growth and development of infants and young children; and that breast-feeding is an important aspect of primary health care;

Considering that when mothers do not breast-feed, or only do so partially, there is a legitimate market for infant formula and for suitable ingredients from which to prepare it; that all these products should accordingly be made accessible to those who need them through commercial or non-commercial distribution systems; and that they should not be marketed or distributed in ways that may interfere with the protection and promotion of breast-feeding;

Recognizing further that inappropriate feeding practices lead to infant malnutrition, morbidity and mortality in all countries, and that improper practices in the marketing of breast-milk substitutes and related products can contribute to these major public health problems;

Convinced that it is important for infants to receive appropriate complementary foods, usually when the infant reaches four to six months of age, and that every effort should be made to use locally available foods; and convinced, nevertheless, that such complementary foods should not be used as breast-milk substitutes;

Appreciating that there are a number of social and economic factors affecting breast-feeding, and that, accordingly, governments should develop social support systems to protect, facilitate and encourage it, and that they should create an environment that fosters breast-feeding, provides appropriate family and community support, and protects mothers from factors that inhibit breast-feeding;

Affirming that health care systems, and the heath professionals and other health workers serving in them, have an essential role to play in guiding infant feeding practices, encouraging and facilitating breast-feeding, and providing objective and consistent advice to mothers and families about the superior value of breast-feeding, or where needed, on the proper use of infant formula, whether manufactured industrially or home-prepared;

Affirming further that educational systems and other social services should be involved in the protection and promotion of breast-feeding, and in the appropriate use of complementary foods;

Aware that families, communities, women's organizations and other nongovernmental organizations have a special role to play in the protection and promotion of breast-feeding and in ensuring the support needed by pregnant women and mothers of infants and young children, whether breast-feeding or not;

Affirming the need for governments, organizations of the United Nations system, nongovernmental organizations, experts in various related disciplines, consumer groups and industry to cooperate in activities aimed at the improvement of maternal, infant and young child health and nutrition;

Recognizing that governments should undertake a variety of health, nutrition and other social measures to promote healthy growth and development of infants and young children, and that this Code concerns only one aspect of these measures;

Considering that manufacturers and distributors of breast-milk substitutes have an important and constructive role to play in relation to infant feeding, and in the promotion of the aim of this Code and its proper implementation;

Affirming that governments are called upon to take action appropriate to their social and legislative framework and their overall development objectives to give effect to the principles and aim of this Code, including the enactment of legislation, regulations or other suitable measures;

Believing that, in the light of the foregoing considerations, and in view of the vulnerability of infants in the early months of life and the risks involved in inappropriate feeding practices, including the unnecessary and improper use of breast-milk substitutes, the marketing of breast-milk substitutes requires special treatment, which makes usual marketing practices unsuitable for these products;

THEREFORE:

The Member States hereby agree the following articles which are recommended as a basis for action.

Reference

1. *International Code of Marketing of Breast-milk Substitutes*, Geneva, World Health Organization, 1981; published by WHO in Arabic, Chinese, English, French, Russian and Spanish.

Article 1
Aim of the Code

The aim of this Code is to contribute to the provision of safe and adequate nutrition for infants, by the protection and promotion of breast-feeding, and by ensuring the proper use of breast-milk substitutes, when these are necessary, on the basis of adequate information and through appropriate marketing and distribution.

Article 2
Scope of the Code

The Code applies to the marketing, and practices related thereto, of the following products: breast-milk substitutes, including infant formula; other milk products, foods and beverages, including bottle-fed complementary foods, when marketed or otherwise represented to be suitable, with or without modification, for use as a partial or total replacement of breast milk; feeding bottle and teats. It also applies to their quality and availability, and to information concerning their use.

Article 3
Definitions

For the purposes of this Code:

"Breast-milk substitute" means any food being marketed or otherwise represented as a partial or total replacement for breast milk, whether or not suitable for that purpose.

"Complementary food" means any food, whether manufactured or locally prepared, suitable as a complement to breast milk or to infant formula, when either becomes insufficient to satisfy the nutritional requirements of the infant. Such food is also commonly called "weaning food" or "breast-milk supplement".

"Container"	means	any form of packaging of products for sale as a normal retail unit, including wrappers.
"Distributor"	means	a person, corporation or any other entity in the public or private sector engaged in the business (whether directly or indirectly) of marketing at the wholesale or retail level a product within the scope of this Code. A "primary distributor" is a manufacturer's sales agent, representative, national distributor or broker.
"Health care system"	means	governmental, nongovernmental or private institutions or organizations engaged, directly or indirectly, in health care for mothers, infants and pregnant women; and nurseries or child-care institutions. It also includes health workers in private practice. For the purposes of this Code, the health care system does not include pharmacies or other established sales outlets.
"Heath worker"	means	a person working in a component of such a health care system, whether professional or non-professional, including voluntary, unpaid workers.
"Infant formula"	means	a breast-milk substitute formulated industrially in accordance with applicable Codex Alimentarius standards, to satisfy the normal nutritional requirements of infants up to between four and six months of age, and adapted to their physiological characteristics. Infant formula may also be prepared at home, in which case it is described as "home-prepared".
"Label"	means	any tag, brand, mark, pictorial or other descriptive matter, written, printed, stencilled, marked, embossed or impressed on, or attached to, a container (see above) of any product within the scope of this Code.
"Manufacturer"	means	a corporation or other entity in the public or private sector engaged in the business or function (whether directly or through an agent or through an entity controlled by or under contract with it) of manufacturing a product within the scope of this Code.

"Marketing"	means	product promotion, distribution, selling, advertising, product public relations, and information services.
"Marketing personnel"	means	any persons whose functions involve the marketing of a product or products coming within the scope of this Code.
"Samples"	means	single or small quantities of a product provided without cost.
"Supplies"	means	quantities of a product provided for use over an extended period, free or at a low price, for social purposes, including those provided to families in need.

Article 4
Information and education

4.1 Governments should have the responsibility to ensure that objective and consistent information is provided on infant and young child feeding for use by families and those involved in the field of infant and young child nutrition. This responsibility should cover either the planning, provision, design and dissemination of information, or their control.

4.2 Informational and educational materials, whether written, audio, or visual, dealing with the feeding of infants and intended to reach pregnant women and mothers of infants and young children, should include information on all the following points: (a) the benefits and superiority of breast-feeding; (b) maternal nutrition, and the preparation for and maintenance of breast-feeding; (c) the negative effect on breast-feeding of introducing partial bottle-feeding; (d) the difficulty of reversing the decision not to breast-feed; and (e) where needed, the proper use of infant formula, whether manufactured industrially or home-prepared. When such materials contain information about the use of infant formula, they should include the social and financial implications of its use; the health hazards of inappropriate foods or feeding methods; and, in particular, the health hazards of unnecessary or improper use of infant formula and other breast-milk substitutes. Such materials should not use any pictures or text which may idealize the use of breast-milk substitutes.

4.3   Donations of informational or educational equipment or materials by manufacturers or distributors should be made only at the request and with the written approval of the appropriate government authority or within guidelines given by governments for this purpose. Such equipment or materials may bear the donating company's name or logo, but should not refer to a proprietary product that is within the scope of this Code, and should be distributed only through the health care system.

Article 5
The general public and mothers

5.1   There should be no advertising or other form of promotion to the general public of products within the scope of this Code.

5.2   Manufacturers and distributors should not provide, directly or indirectly, to pregnant women, mothers or members of their families, samples of products within the scope of this Code.

5.3   In conformity with paragraphs 1 and 2 of this Article, there should be no point-of-sale advertising, giving of samples, or any other promotion device to induce sales directly to the consumer at the retail level, such as special displays, discount coupons, premiums, special sales, loss-leaders and tie-in sales, for products within the scope of this Code. This provision should not restrict the establishment of pricing policies and practices intended to provide products at lower prices on a long-term basis.

5.4   Manufacturers and distributors should not distribute to pregnant women or mothers of infants and young children any gifts of articles or utensils which may promote the use of breast-milk substitutes or bottle-feeding.

5.5   Marketing personnel, in their business capacity, should not seek direct or indirect contact of any kind with pregnant women or with mothers of infants and young children.

Article 6
Health care systems

6.1 The health authorities in Member States should take appropriate measures to encourage and protect breast-feeding and promote the principles of this Code, and should give appropriate information and advice to health workers in regard to their responsibilities, including the information specified in Article 4.2.

6.2 No facility of a health care system should be used for the purpose of promoting infant formula or other products within the scope of this Code. This Code does not, however, preclude the dissemination of information to health professionals as provided in Article 7.2.

6.3 Facilities of health care systems should not be used for the display of products within the scope of this Code, for placards or posters concerning such products, or for the distribution of material provided by a manufacturer or distributor other than that specified in Article 4.3.

6.4 The use by the health care system of "professional services representatives", "mothercraft nurses" or similar personnel, provided or paid for by manufacturers or distributors, should not be permitted.

6.5 Feeding with infant formula, whether manufactured or home-prepared, should be demonstrated only by health workers, or other community workers if necessary; and only to the mothers or family members who need to use it; and the information given should include a clear explanation of the hazards of improper use.

6.6 Donations or low-price sales to institutions or organizations of supplies of infant formula or other products within the scope of this Code, whether for use in the institutions or for distribution outside them, may be made. Such supplies should only be used or distributed for infants who have to be fed on breast-milk substitutes. If these supplies are distributed for use outside the institutions, this should be done only by the institutions or organizations concerned. Such donations or low-price sales should not be used by manufacturers or distributors as a sales inducement.

6.7 Where donated supplies of infant formula or other products within the scope of this Code are distributed outside an institution, the institution or organization should take steps to ensure that supplies can be continued as long as the infants concerned need them. Donors, as well as institutions or organizations concerned, should bear in mind this responsibility.

6.8   Equipment and materials, in addition to those referred to in Article 4.3, donated to a health care system may bear a company's name or logo, but should not refer to any proprietary product within the scope of this Code.

Article 7
Health workers

7.1   Health workers should encourage and protect breast-feeding; and those who are concerned in particular with maternal and infant nutrition should make themselves familiar with their responsibilities under this Code, including the information specified in Article 4.2.

7.2   Information provided by manufacturers and distributors to health professionals regarding products within the scope of this Code should be restricted to scientific and factual matters, and such information should not imply or create a belief that bottle-feeding is equivalent or superior to breast-feeding. It should also include the information specified in Article 4.2.

7.3   No financial or material inducements to promote products within the scope of this Code should be offered by manufacturers or distributors to health workers or members of their families, nor should these be accepted by health workers or members of their families.

7.4   Samples of infant formula or other products within the scope of this Code, or of equipment or utensils for their preparation or use, should not be provided to health workers except when necessary for the purpose of professional evaluation or research at the institutional level. Health workers should not give samples of infant formula to pregnant women, mothers of infants and young children, or members of their families.

7.5   Manufacturers and distributors of products within the scope of this Code should disclose to the institution to which a recipient health worker is affiliated any contribution made to him or on his behalf for fellowships, study tours, research grants, attendance at professional conferences, or the like. Similar disclosures should be made by the recipient.

Article 8
Persons employed by manufacturers and distributors

8.1   In systems of sales incentives for marketing personnel, the volume of sales of products within the scope of this Code should not be included in the calculation of bonuses, nor should quotas be set specifically for sales of these products. This should not be understood to prevent the payment of bonuses based on the overall sales by a company of other products marketed by it.

8.2   Personnel employed in marketing products within the scope of this Code should not, as part of their job responsibilities, perform educational functions in relation to pregnant women or mothers of infants and young children. This should not be understood as preventing such personnel from being used for other functions by the health care system at the request and with the written approval of the appropriate authority of the government concerned.

Article 9
Labelling

9.1   Labels should be designed to provide the necessary information about the appropriate use of the product, and so as not to discourage breast-feeding.

9.2   Manufacturers and distributors of infant formula should ensure that each container has a clear, conspicuous, and easily readable and understandable message printed on it, or on a label which cannot readily become separated from it, in an appropriate language, which includes all the following points: (a) the words "Important Notice" or their equivalent; (b) a statement of the superiority of breast-feeding; (c) a statement that the product should be used only on the advice of a health worker as to the need for its use and the proper method of use; (d) instructions for appropriate preparation, and a warning against the health hazards of inappropriate preparation. Neither the container nor the label should have pictures of infants, nor should they have other pictures or texts which may idealize the use of infant formula. They may, however, have graphics for easy identification of the product as a breast-milk substitute and for illustrating methods of preparation. The terms "humanized", "maternalized" or similar terms should not be used. Inserts giving additional information about the product and its proper use, subject to the above conditions, may be included in the package or retail unit. When labels give instructions for modifying a product into infant formula, the above should apply.

9.3 Food products within the scope of this Code, marketed for infant feeding, which do not meet all the requirements of an infant formula, but which can be modified to do so, should carry on the label a warning that the unmodified product should not be the sole source of nourishment of an infant. Since sweetened condensed milk·is not suitable for infant feeding, nor for use as a main ingredient of infant formula, its label should not contain purported instructions on how to modify it for that purpose.

9.4 The label of food products within the scope of this Code should also state all the following points: (a) the ingredients used; (b) the composition/analysis of the product; (c) the storage conditions required; and (d) the batch number and the date before which the product is to be consumed, taking into account the climatic and storage conditions of the country concerned.

Article 10
Quality

10.1 The quality of products is an essential element for the protection of the health of infants and therefore should be of a high recognized standard.

10.2 Food products within the scope of this Code should, when sold or otherwise distributed, meet applicable standards recommended by the Codex Alimentarius Commission and also the Codex Code of Hygienic Practice for Foods for Infants and Children.

Article 11
Implementation and monitoring

11.1 Governments should take action to give effect to the principles and aim of this Code, as appropriate to their social and legislative framework, including the adoption of national legislation, regulations or other suitable measures. For this purpose, governments should seek, when necessary, the cooperation of WHO, UNICEF and other agencies of the United Nations system. National policies and measures, including laws and regulations, which are adopted to give effect to the principles and aim of this Code should be publicly stated, and should apply on the same basis to all those involved in the manufacture and marketing of products within the scope of this Code.

11.2 Monitoring the application of this Code lies with governments acting individually, and collectively through the World Health Organization as provided in paragraphs 6 and 7 of this Article. The manufacturers and distributors of products within the scope of this Code, and appropriate nongovernmental organizations, professional groups, and consumer organizations should collaborate with governments to this end.

11.3 Independently of any other measures taken for implementation of this Code, manufacturers and distributors of products within the scope of this Code should regard themselves as responsible for monitoring their marketing practices according to the principles and aim of this Code, and for taking steps to ensure that their conduct at every level conforms to them.

11.4 Nongovernmental organizations, professional groups, institutions, and individuals concerned should have the responsibility of drawing the attention of manufacturers or distributors to activities which are incompatible with the principles and aim of this Code, so that appropriate action can be taken. The appropriate governmental authority should also be informed.

11.5 Manufacturers and primary distributors of products within the scope of this Code should apprise each member of their marketing personnel of the Code and of their responsibilities under it.

11.6 In accordance with Article 62 of the Constitution of the World Health Organization, Member States shall communicate annually to the Director-General information on action taken to give effect to the principles and aim of this Code.

11.7 The Director-General shall report in even years to the World Health Assembly on the status of implementation of the Code; and shall, on request, provide technical support to Member States preparing national legislation or regulations, or taking other appropriate measures in implementation and furtherance of the principles and aim of this Code.

Resolutions of the World Health Assembly with particular reference to the International Code of Marketing of Breast-milk Substitutes

WHA39.28 Infant and young child feeding

The Thirty-ninth World Health Assembly,

Recalling resolutions WHA27.43, WHA31.47, WHA33.32, WHA34.22, WHA35.26 and WHA37.30 which dealt with infant and young child feeding;

Having considered the progress and evaluation report by the Director-General on infant and young child nutrition (1);

Recognizing that the implementation of the International Code of Marketing of Breast-milk Substitutes is an important contribution to healthy infant and young child feeding in all countries;

Aware that today, five years after the adoption of the International Code, many Member States have made substantial efforts to implement it, but that many products unsuitable for infant feeding are none the less being promoted and used for this purpose; and that sustained and concerted efforts will therefore continue to be necessary to achieve full implementation of and compliance with the International Code as well as the cessation of the marketing of unsuitable products and the improper promotion of breast-milk substitutes;

Noting with great satisfaction the guidelines concerning the main health and socioeconomic circumstances in which infants have to be fed on breast-milk substitutes (2), in the context of Article 6, paragraph 6, of the International Code;

Noting further the statement in the guidelines, paragraph 47: "Since the large majority of infants born in maternity wards and hospitals are full term, they require no nourishment other than colostrum during their first 24-48 hours of life — the amount of time often spent by a mother and her infant in such an institutional setting. Only small quantities of breast-milk substitutes are ordinarily required to meet the needs of a minority of infants in these facilities, and they should only be available in ways that do not interfere with the protection and promotion of breast-feeding for the majority";

1. ENDORSES the report of the Director-General (1);

2.   URGES Member States:

(1)   to implement the Code if they have not yet done so;

(2)   to ensure that the practices and procedures of their health care systems are consistent with the principles and aim of the International Code;

(3)   to make the fullest use of all concerned parties — health professional bodies, nongovernmental organizations, consumer organizations, manufacturers and distributors — generally, in protecting and promoting breast-feeding and, specifically, in implementing the Code and monitoring its implementation and compliance with its provisions;

(4)   to seek the cooperation of manufacturers and distributors of products within the scope of Article 2 of the Code, in providing all information considered necessary for monitoring the implementation of the Code;

(5)   to provide the Director-General with complete and detailed information on the implementation of the Code;

(6)   to ensure that the small amounts of breast-milk substitutes needed for the minority of infants who require them in maternity wards and hospitals are made available through the normal procurement channels and not through free or subsidized supplies;

3.   REQUESTS the Director-General:

(1)   to propose a simplified and standardized form for use by Member States to facilitate the monitoring and evaluation by them of their implementation of the Code and reporting thereon to WHO, as well as the preparation by WHO of a consolidated report covering each of the articles of the Code;

(2)   to specifically direct the attention of Member States and other interested parties to the following:

(a)   any food or drink given before complementary feeding is nutritionally required may interfere with the initiation or maintenance of breast-feeding and therefore should neither be promoted nor encouraged for use by infants during this period;

(b)   the practice being introduced in some countries of providing infants with specially formulated milks (so-called "follow-up milks") is not necessary.

May 1986   WHA39/1986/REC/1, 29

References

1. Document WHA39/1986/REC/1, p. 102.
2. Document WHA39/1986/REC/1, p. 122.

WHA47.5 Infant and young child nutrition

The Forty-seventh World Health Assembly,

Having considered the report by the Director-General on infant and young child nutrition (1);

Recalling resolutions WHA33.32, WHA34.22, WHA35.26, WHA37.30, WHA39.28, WHA41.11, WHA43.3, WHA45.34 and WHA46.7 concerning infant and young child nutrition, appropriate feeding practices and related questions;

Reaffirming its support for all these resolutions and reiterating the recommendations to Member States contained therein;

Bearing in mind the superiority of breast milk as the biological norm for the nourishment of infants, and that a deviation from this norm is associated with increased risks to the health of infants and mothers,

1.   THANKS the Director-General for his report;

2.   URGES Member States to take the following measures:

  (1)   to promote sound infant and young child nutrition, in keeping with their commitment to the World Declaration and Plan of Action for Nutrition (2), through coherent effective intersectoral action, including:

  (a)   increasing awareness among health personnel, nongovernmental organizations, communities and the general public of the importance of breast-feeding and its superiority to any other infant feeding method;

  (b)   supporting mothers in their choice to breast-feed by removing obstacles and preventing interference that they may face in health services, the workplace, or the community;

  (c)   ensuring that all health personnel concerned are trained in appropriate infant and young child feeding practices, including the application of the principles laid down in the joint WHO/UNICEF statement of breast-feeding and the role of maternity services (3);

  (d)   fostering appropriate complementary feeding practices from the age of about six months, emphasizing continued breast-feeding and frequent feeding with safe and adequate amounts of local foods;

(2)   to ensure that there are no donations of free or subsidized supplies of breast-milk substitutes and other products covered by the International Code of Marketing of Breast-milk Substitutes in any part of the health care system;

(3)   to exercise extreme caution when planning, implementing or supporting emergency relief operations, by protecting, promoting and supporting breast-feeding for infants, and ensuring that donated supplies of breast-milk substitutes or other products covered by the scope of the International Code are given only if all the following conditions apply:

(a)   infants have to be fed on breast-milk substitutes, as outlined in the guidelines concerning the main health and socioeconomic circumstances in which infants have to be fed on breast-milk substitutes (4);

(b)   the supply is continued for as long as the infants concerned need it;

(c)   the supply is not used as a sales inducement;

(4)   to inform the labour sector, and employers' and workers' organizations, about the multiple benefits of breast-feeding for infants and mothers, and the implications for maternity protection in the workplace;

3.   REQUESTS the Director-General:

(1)   to use his good offices for cooperation with all parties concerned in giving effect to this and related resolutions of the Health Assembly in their entirety;

(2)   to complete development of a comprehensive global approach and programme of action to strengthen national capacities for improving infant and young child feeding practices, including the development of methods and criteria for national assessment of breast-feeding trends and practices;

(3)   to support Member States, at their request, in monitoring infant and young chid feeding practices and trends in health facilities and households, in keeping with new standard breast-feeding indicators;

(4)   to urge Member States to join in the Baby-friendly Hospital Initiative and to support them, at their request, in implementing this Initiative, particularly in their efforts to improve educational curricula and in-service training for all health and administrative personnel concerned;

(5)   to increase and strengthen support to Member States, at their request, in giving effect to the principles and aim of the International Code and all relevant resolutions, and to advise Member States on a framework which they may use in monitoring their application, as appropriate to national circumstances;

(6)   to develop, in consultation with other concerned parties and as part of WHO's normative function, guiding principles for the use in emergency situations of breast-milk substitutes or other products covered by the International Code which the competent authorities in Member States may use, in the light of national circumstances, to ensure the optimal infant-feeding conditions;

(7)   to complete, in cooperation with selected research institutions, collection of revised reference data and the preparation of guidelines for their use and interpretation, so as to assess the growth of breast-fed infants;

(8)   to seek additional technical and financial resources for intensifying WHO's support to Member States in infant feeding and in the implementation of the International Code and subsequent relevant resolutions.

Hbk Res., Vol. III (3rd ed.), 1.12.1

(Eleventh plenary meeting, 9 May 1994 -

Committee A, first report)

References

1. Document WHA47/1994/REC/1. Annex 1.

2. *World Declaration and Plan of Action for Nutrition.* FAO/WHO, International Conference on Nutrition, Rome, December 1992.

3. *Protecting, promoting and supporting breast-feeding: the special role of maternity services.* A joint WHO/UNICEF statement. Geneva, World Health Organization, 1989.

4. Document WHA39/1986/REC/1, Annex 6, part 2.

In-depth review and evaluation of national action taken to give effect to the International Code of Marketing of Breast-milk Substitutes recommendations of a technical meeting (1)

The Hague, 30 September–3 October 1991

In 1990 the Forty-third World Health Assembly, by resolution WHA43.3 (2), requested the Director-General "to support Member States ... in adopting measures to improve infant and young child nutrition, *inter alia* by collecting and disseminating information on relevant national action of interest to all Member States". With funds provided by the Government of the Netherlands, and in collaboration with the Government of Sweden and the Swedish International Development Authority, WHO provided technical and other support to 14 Member States (3) that had indicated their desire to undertake an in-depth review and evaluation of their own experiences in giving effect to the International Code, using a common review and evaluation framework (CREF) (4).

The results of the 14-country exercise were summarized in a background document, which served as the basis for discussion by representatives of the countries concerned at a technical meeting on the subject held in The Hague, with UNICEF participation, from 30 September to 3 October 1991. The purpose of the meeting was to consider in concrete and practical terms what Member States can do to give effect to the principles and aim of the International Code, with support from WHO, UNICEF and other interested parties. Also present at the meeting were representatives of five nongovernmental organizations in official relations with WHO that have a particular interest in infant feeding: the International Federation of Gynaecology and Obstetrics, the International Pediatric Association, the International Confederation of Midwives, the International Organization of Consumers Unions (Consumers International), and the International Association of Infant Food Manufacturers.

Participants were unanimous in observing that their national review and evaluation exercise had been valuable in terms of increasing awareness and understanding of the importance of the International Code and its place in their countries; they considered that all countries would benefit from such an exercise.

The report of the technical meeting includes, in addition to the background document, a summary of the discussions, and a number of conclusions and recommendations, drawn up on the basis of lessons learned.

The recommendations under the heading **development and implementation** were as follows:

- Governments should make a political commitment to give effect to the principles and aim of the International Code **in its entirety**, as a minimum measure. Political commitment implies monitoring of compliance with national measures, imposition of sanctions, and availability of adequate material and human resources to follow up.

- Governments have full responsibility for formulating and adopting national measures to give effect to the International Code. In so doing, however, they should consult all concerned parties as an important means of ensuring their active participation in the implementation of the measures.

- When adopting measures to give effect to the International Code, national authorities should use clear definitions and exact specifications. The scope of these measures should include all products that are perceived and used as breast-milk substitutes, whether or not suitable for this purpose, and whatever the age of the children concerned (5). When appropriate, technical support in this regard should be sought from WHO.

- National measures adopted to give effect to the International Code should be seen as a standard component of every maternal and child health policy and programme. They should apply to health services in both the public and the private sector.

- The competent national authorities, where this has not already been done, should appoint a national breast-feeding coordinator and establish a multisectoral breast-feeding committee composed of concerned parties. The responsibilities of the coordinator and of the committee should include ensuring observance of national measures taken to give effect to the International Code.

- International organizations, directly or through their country offices where they exist, should provide national authorities with information concerning the International Code. Documentation on measures that have been adopted in various countries, together with information on experience in their implementation that could be useful to other countries, should be gathered and disseminated by WHO, UNICEF, the Code documentation centre (6), and other appropriate organizations and bodies.

- Steps currently being taken towards ending the donation or low-price sale of samples of infant formulas to maternity wards and hospitals should be continued and strengthened. Henceforth, infant formulas should be made available through the normal procurement channels in **all** countries and not through free or subsidized supplies.

- Charitable and other donor agencies should exert great care in initiating, or responding to, requests for free supplies of infant foods. These agencies should review, and adapt as appropriate, the policies relating to the distribution and use of milk products for infant feeding that have been adopted by such bodies as the Office of the High Commissioner for Refugees, the World Food Programme, and the International Committee of the Red Cross. In order to avoid interfering with breast-feeding, no more than the minimum required amounts of infant foods should be provided for distribution under appropriate supervision and follow-up.

- Consultations should be held regarding the problem of countries that, owing to newly evolving market situations, are particularly vulnerable to marketing practices relating to products within the scope of the International Code. This includes countries that are in the process of moving from centrally planned to market economies and to countries with population groups that are beginning to participate in a cash economy.

Recommendations for **training and education in the health sector** were as follows:

- National measures which have been adopted to give effect to the International Code should be presented in clear and understandable language, and disseminated widely.

- All initial and in-service health worker training in breast-feeding should include: (a) information and advice regarding the responsibilities of health workers under the national measures adopted to give effect to the International Code; (b) discussion of the principles summarized, and operational targets contained, in the Innocenti Declaration (7) and the joint WHO/UNICEF statement on breast-feeding and maternity services (8); and (c) information on lactation management and on means of fostering the establishment of breast-feeding support groups in the community.

- WHO should encourage and support the revision and, where necessary, the preparation of the parts of health workers' training curricula, textbooks and other learning materials relating to infant feeding, in association with relevant

International professional and voluntary organizations. These materials should state the principles and aim of the International Code and give information in regard to health workers' responsibilities under it.

- On behalf of their membership in countries, international professional associations should develop, or where appropriate strengthen, guidelines for establishing ethical standards of conduct for health workers and manufacturers and distributors of products within the scope of the International Code.

Recommendations concerning **information to the general public and mothers** were as follows:

- National authorities should provide information and education on infant and young child nutrition and feeding that is adapted to local language, culture, and literacy.

- Governments should explore, on a bilateral or multilateral basis, means of regulating the promotion via international satellite and cable television transmission of products within the scope of the International Code, in keeping with the Code's provisions.

- WHO should continue to provide appropriate learning materials, include video films, on infant and young child nutrition and feeding, for adaptation and use in countries.

- The feeding bottle and teat should not be used as a child-care symbol (9), nor should it be used in connection with promoting any other products, e.g. mineral water and baby-care items.

Recommendations for **monitoring and enforcement** were as follows:

- To the extent possible, the monitoring of national measures adopted to give effect to the International Code should be undertaken through existing mechanisms, e.g. those relating to food inspection, health service practices, and trade regulation. Appropriate training should be provided for those persons concerned.

- The monitoring of national measures should include periodic surveys of knowledge, attitudes and practices among health workers.

- WHO, in collaboration with other agencies and organizations, should develop indicators, based on agree definitions, for monitoring national measures. These indicators, together with guidelines for their adoption and use, should be disseminated to countries.

The following recommendations were addressed to **manufactures and distributors** of products within the scope of the International Code:

- Manufacturers and distributors of **all** products within the scope of the International Code should comply with the Code **in its entirety in all countries**, (10) unless specifically prohibited from doing so by national legislation (11).

- Governments and concerned organizations should seek to define and adopt internationally recognized standards relating to the design and quality of feeding bottles and teats.

- At the retain level, infant formulas displayed for sale should be separated from other products (e.g. herbal teas, starchy gruels, sweetened condensed milk, and follow-up formulas) commonly used for infant feeding.

References

1. The full report of the meeting is contained in document WHO/NUT/MCH/91.2. The meeting recommendations reproduced here also appeared in the report by the Director-General to the Forty-fifth (1992) World Health Assembly on infant and young child nutrition, which appears in document WHA45/1992/REC/1, Annex 9, pp. 230-232.

2. *Handbook of resolutions and decisions*, Vol. III, 1993, pp. 63-64.

3. Brazil, Egypt, Finland, Guatemala, Islamic Republic of Iran, Kenya, the Netherlands, Nigeria, Papua New Guinea, the Philippines, Poland, Sweden, United Kingdom of Great Britain and Northern Ireland, and Yemen.

4. *The review and evaluation of national action taken to give effect to the aim and principles of the International Code of Marketing of Breast-milk Substitutes. A common review and evaluation framework (CREF).* Informal document prepared by the Nutrition and Maternal and Child Health and Family Planning Programmes, Geneva, World Health Organization, 1991.

5. The report by the Director-General on infant and young child nutrition to the Forty-fifth World Health Assembly (1992) noted that "the representative of the International Association of Infant Food Manufacturers (IFM)[a member body of the International Special Dietary Foods Industries, an international nongovernmental organization in official relations with WHO since 1987], at the meeting in The Hague ... said that she had taken careful note of the concerns expressed by some governments and other parties about the potentially negative consequences for child health that could result from confusion in the market place between *bona fide* infant formula and follow-up formula. She indicated that these concerns would be brought to the attention of IFM members, with a view to their taking all necessary steps to ensure that their marketing practices made a very clear distinction between these two products" (document WHA45/1992/REC/1, Annex 9, paragraph 51).

6. The International Baby Food Action Network (IBFAN), in Penang, Malaysia, is located in the Regional Office for Asia and the Pacific of the International Organization of Consumers Unions (Consumers International), which is a nongovernmental organization admitted into official relations with WHO in 1986. IBFAN periodically holds training courses on implementing the International Code for participants from various countries, who are sponsored by governments or with private funds. Courses cover policy and socioeconomic and legal aspects of the Code, and individual guidance and references are provided. Participants also have access to the extensive range of related material collected by the Code documentation centre on the premises.

7. A meeting of government policy-makers from over 30 developed and developing countries (Florence, July 1990) adopted the Innocenti Declaration on the Protection, Promotion and Support of Breastfeeding. The Forty-fifth World Health Assembly (1992), in resolution WHA45.34, urged Member States to give full expression to the Declaration's operational targets, namely that, by 1995, (a) all governments should have appointed a national breast-feeding coordinator and established a multisectoral breast-feeding committee; (b) ensured that every facility providing maternity services applies the principles laid down in the joint WHO/UNICEF statement on the subject; (c) taken action to give effect to the principles and aim of the International Code; and (d) enacted legislation, and adopted means for its enforcement, to protect breast-feeding rights of working women.

8. *Protecting, promoting and supporting breast-feeding: the special role of maternity services, op. cit.*

9. Following the meeting, the representatives of the International Organization of Consumers Unions and the President of the International Association of Infant Food Manufacturers wrote, respectively, to the International Organization for Standardization (ISO) and to the International Air Transport Association (IATA) to recommend that a suitable child-care symbol be found to replace the feeding bottle frequently used in public transport facilities and to offer their cooperation to this end. Both ISO and IATA are nongovernmental organizations in official relations with WHO.

10. Manufacturers and distributors of products within the scope of the International Code frequently make a distinction between developing and industrialized countries where their marketing practices in relation to the Code are concerned. However, neither the Code itself nor the World Health Assembly has made such a distinction.

11. In October 1989, IFM "reaffirmed to the WHO Director-General the commitment of its member companies to support the principles and aim of the WHO Code. In practice, this individual, voluntary commitment by member companies is carried out by conforming to the WHO Code in its entirety in developing countries, except where specific national codes or other measures have been implemented by governments. In developed countries, IFM companies comply with the national codes and regulations, and/or with voluntary industry codes established in consultation with the relevant authorities. Such voluntary codes are designed to give practical effect to the WHO Code as appropriate to the social and legislative framework of the countries concerned. In their absence, each company remains responsible for the marketing practices best suited to consumer needs, in line with the aim of the WHO Code, and in accordance with the circumstances and applicable legal requirements in any specific country". Source: *IFM: a commitment to infant and young child health*, Paris, 1991, pp. 15–16.

Suggested frameworks

Annex 4
Suggested framework for assessing informational and educational
materials intended to reach mothers and the general public 61

Annex 5
Suggested framework for assessing informational materials about infant
formula provided to, or for the use of, health professionals 65

Annex 6
Suggested framework for assessing the adequacy of labels
on products within the scope of the Code 67

Annex 7
Suggested framework for conducting site visits 73

Suggested framework for assessing informational and educational materials intended to reach mothers and the general public (1)

(Article 4 of the International Code)

Ideally, the answer to every question will be "yes".
Does the audiovisual or written material satisfy the following criteria?

Is clear information provided on the benefits and superiority of breast-feeding?	Yes / No
Is clear information provided on maternal nutrition?	Yes / No
Is clear information provided on preparation for and maintenance of breast-feeding?	Yes / No
Is clear information provided on the negative effect on breast-feeding of introducing partial bottle-feeding?	Yes / No
Is clear information provided on the difficulty of reversing the decision not to breast-feed?	Yes / No
Is clear information provided, where needed, on the proper use of infant formula?	Yes / No
When information on the use of infant formula is provided:	
• Does it include information on the social and financial implications of using infant formula?	Yes / No
• Does it include information on the health hazards of inappropriate foods or feeding methods?	Yes / No
• Does it include information on the health hazards of unnecessary or improper use of infant formula?	Yes / No
Absence of pictures which idealize the use of infant formula?	Yes / No
Absence of text which idealizes the use of infant formula?	Yes / No
No advertising or promotion of infant formula (Article 5)?	Yes / No

Bearing the donating company's name or logo **only**?	Yes / No
Absence of any reference to a proprietary product within the scope of the Code?	Yes / No
The material, if from a manufacturer or distributor, has been donated only at the request and with the written approval of the competent government authority or within guidelines given for this purpose?	Yes / No
The material has been distributed only through the health care system?	Yes / No
Does the material comply with the aim of the Code which is to contribute to the provision of safe and adequate nutrition for infants:	
• By protecting and promoting breast-feeding?	Yes / No
• Ensuring the proper use of breast-milk substitutes, when they are necessary, on the basis of adequate information and through appropriate marketing and distribution?	Yes / No
• Are donations of materials made only at the request and with the written approval of the competent authority or within guidelines the authority has established?	Yes / No

Reference

1. For materials intended for health workers, see Annex 5.

Suggested framework for assessing data on informational materials intended to reach mothers and the general public	Fully complies	Complies, but with mixed messages	Does not comply	Requirement not applicable or not known
Clear information on the benefits and superiority of breast-feeding Clear information on maternal nutrition.				
Clear information on preparation for and maintenance of breast-feeding. Clear information on the negative effect on breast-feeding of introducing partial bottle-feeding. Clear information on the difficulty of reversing the decision not to breast-feed. Clear information, where needed, on the proper use of formula. When information on the use of formula is provided it includes information on:				
• The social and financial implications of using formula.				
• The health hazards of inappropriate foods or feeding methods.				
• The health hazards of unnecessary or improper use of infant formula.				
Absence of pictures which may idealize the use of infant formula				
Absence of text which may idealize the use of infant formula.				
Infant formula not advertised or promoted in any way (Article 5).				
Donated equipment or materials bearing the donating company's name or logo **only**.				

Suggested framework for assessing data on informational materials intended to reach mothers and the general public	Fully complies	Complies, but with mixed messages	Does not comply	Requirement not applicable or not known
Absence of any reference to a proprietary product within the scope of the Code. Donated only at the request of, or with the approval of, the competent authority. Complies with written guidelines Distributed **only** through the health care system. Material complies with the aim of the Code which is to contribute to the provision of safe and adequate nutrition for infants: • By protecting and promoting breast-feeding, and • Ensuring the proper use of breast-milk substitutes, when they are necessary, on the basis of adequate information and through appropriate marketing and distribution.				

Suggested framework for assessing informational materials about infant formula provided by manufacturers of distributors to, or for the use of, health professionals (1)

(Article 7 of the International Code)

Ideally, the answer to every question will be "yes".
Does the video or document satisfy all the following criteria?

Is this material intended only for the use of health professionals?	Yes / No
Is the information restricted to scientific and factual matters?	Yes / No
Does the information reflect current knowledge and responsible opinion?	Yes / No
Is clear information provided on the benefits and superiority of breast-feeding?	Yes / No
Is clear information provided on maternal nutrition?	Yes / No
Is clear information provided on preparation for and maintenance of breast-feeding?	Yes / No
Is clear information provided on the negative effect on breast-feeding of introducing partial bottle-feeding?	Yes / No
Is clear information provided on the difficulty of reversing the decision not to breast-feed?	Yes / No
Is clear information provided, where needed, on the proper use of formula?	Yes / No
When information on the use of formula is provided:	
• Does it include information on the social and financial implications of using infant formula?	Yes / No
• Does it include information on the health hazards of inappropriate foods or feeding methods?	Yes / No

• Does it include information on the health hazards of unnecessary or improper use of infant formula?	Yes / No
Absence of pictures which idealize the use of infant formula?	Yes / No
Absence of text which idealizes the use of infant formula?	Yes / No
Is the material clearly identified with:	
• The name of the manufacturer or importer?	Yes / No
• The date of publication?	Yes / No
Does the distribution of this material avoid any advertising or promotion to the general public (Article 5) of products within the scope of the International Code?	Yes / No
Does the material comply with the aim of the Code, which is to contribute to the provision of safe and adequate nutrition for infants:	
• by protecting and promoting breast-feeding?	Yes / No
• ensuring the proper use of breast-milk substitutes, when they are necessary, on the basis of adequate information and through appropriate marketing and distribution?	Yes / No

Reference

1. For materials intended for mothers and the general public, see Annex 4.

Suggested framework for assessing the adequacy of labels on products within the scope of the Code (Article 9)	Fully complies	Complies, but with mixed messages	Does not comply	Requirement not applicable or not known
Provides the necessary information about the appropriate use of the product, and so as not to discourage breast-feeding. Product identifiable as suitable for infant feeding (may include suitable graphics).				
The specified information is: • Printed on the container or a well-attached label. • Clear and conspicuous. • Easily readable (including inserts). • In an appropriate language.				
The specified information includes: • The words "Important Notice" or their equivalent. • A statement of the superiority of breast-feeding. • A statement that the product should be used only on the advice of a health worker. • Statement on the need for health worker advice on the indications for use. • A statement on the need for health worker advice on the proper method of use.				
There are clear instructions for appropriate preparation (may include graphics). There is a warning against the health hazards of inappropriate preparation.				

Suggested framework for assessing the adequacy of labels on products within the scope of the Code (Article 9)	Fully complies	Complies, but with mixed messages	Does not comply	Requirement not applicable or not known
The label includes:				
• No pictures of infants.				
• No pictures or text which may idealize the use of infant formula.				
• No terms such as "humanized" or "maternalized".				
• A list of the ingredients.				
• The composition/analysis of the product.				
• The storage conditions required.				
• The date before which the product is to be consumed, taking local conditions into account.				
For products marketed for infant feeding, subject to modification, does the label also include:				
• Instructions for modifying the product?				
• A warning that the unmodified product should not be used as the sole source of nourishment?				
PRODUCTS WITHIN THE SCOPE OF THE CODE				
Does the label provide the necessary information about the appropriate use of the product, and so as not to discourage breast-feeding?				

Suggested framework for assessing the adequacy of labels on products within the scope of the Code (Article 9)	Fully complies	Complies, but with mixed messages	Does not comply	Requirement not applicable or not known
Does the specific information include:				
• The words "Important Notice" or their equivalent?				
• A statement that the product should be used only on the advice of a health worker?				
• A statement on the need for health worker advice as to the need for its use?				
• A statement on the need for health worker advice on the proper method of use?				
Are there clear instructions for appropriate preparation (may include graphics)?				
Is there a warning against the health hazards of inappropriate preparation?				
Does the container or label exclude:				
• Pictures of infants?				
• Picture of text which may idealize the use of infant formula?				
• Terms such as "humanized" or "maternalized"?				
Does the container or label include:				
• A list of the ingredients used?				
• The composition/analysis of the product?				
• The storage conditions required?				
• The batch number?				

Suggested framework for assessing the adequacy of labels on products within the scope of the Code (Article 9)	Fully complies	Complies, but with mixed messages	Does not comply	Requirement not applicable or not known
• The date before which the product is to be consumed, taking local climatic and storage conditions into account?				
PRODUCTS MARKETED FOR INFANT FEEDING SUBJECT TO MODIFICATION				
Do these products also include:				
• Instructions for modifying the product to meet the nutritional needs of an infant?				
• A warning that the unmodified product should not be the sole source of nourishment?				
N.B. Products which are not suitable for infant feeding or for modification for infant feeding should not contain purported instructions for feeding to infants.				
Information restricted to scientific and factual matters.				
Information reflects current knowledge and responsible opinion.				
Information avoids implying or creating a belief that bottle-feeding is equivalent or superior to breast-feeding.				
Clear information on the benefits and superiority of breast-feeding.				
Clear information on maternal nutrition.				

Suggested framework for assessing the adequacy of labels on products within the scope of the Code (Article 9)	Fully complies	Complies, but with mixed messages	Does not comply	Requirement not applicable or not known
Clear information on preparation for and maintenance of breast-feeding.				
Clear information on the negative effect on breast-feeding of introducing partial bottle-feeding.				
Clear information on the difficulty of reversing the decision not to breast-feed.				
Clear information, where needed, on the proper use of formula.				
When information on the use of formula is provided it includes information on:				
• The social and financial implications of using formula.				
• The health hazards of inappropriate foods or feeding methods.				
• The health hazards of unnecessary or improper use of infant formula.				
Absence of pictures which may idealize the use of infant formula.				
Absence of text which may idealize the use of infant formula.				
Material clearly identified with:				
• The name of the manufacturer or importer.				
• The brand name/s of the infant formula/s.				
• The date of publication.				

Suggested framework for assessing the adequacy of labels on products within the scope of the Code (Article 9)	**Fully complies**	**Complies, but with mixed messages**	**Does not comply**	**Requirement not applicable or not known**
The distribution of the material avoids advertising or promotion to the general public (Article 5) of products within the scope of the Code (Article 2).				

Suggested framework for conducting site visits, including hospitals, clinics, and other health care facilities

(e.g. immunization clinics, and well-baby/growth monitoring clinics)

- Evidence of measures which protect and promote breast-feeding (e.g. degree to which the "Ten steps to successful breast-feeding" (1) have been implemented or whether facility has achieved "baby-friendly" status).

- Note whether there are copies available of national texts adopted to give effect to the International Code.

- Team members should ask to see equipment or materials which companies have donated whether for use in the facility or for distribution to mothers and families.

- Note whether cans of infant formula, bottles or other items that carry proprietary names are visible, especially in waiting rooms and in rooms where clients receive services.

- Does the facility encourage in any way the use of products within the scope of the Code?

- Look for posters, gifts to mothers, product samples, educational materials (print, audio and video) produced or sponsored by manufacturers or distributors of products within the scope of the International Code, special displays, fliers, pamphlets and any other form of advertising or marketing.

- If hospital discharge packs are given to mothers, note whether they contain any products within the scope of the Code or materials which advertise or promote the use of any of these products.

- Does any equipment or do any materials donated to the health care system by manufacturers and distributors of products within the scope of the Code bear more than a company's name or logo? Is there any mention of, or reference to, a product within the scope of the Code?

- Ask different categories of health workers to provide examples of pamphlets, posters, equipment, information or products given to them by manufacturers.

- Note any differences in marketing and/or breast-feeding practices between public- and private-sector facilities visited.

Retail outlets (e.g. pharmacies, supermarkets, toy stores, small retail outlets)

- What products are on display or otherwise marketed for infant feeding (e.g. infant formula, feeding bottles and teats, baby juices, herbal teas, complementary foods, etc.)?

- Which of these products are covered by the national measures adopted to give effect to the International Code?

- Are there products not covered by the national measures?

- Do all infant feeding products comply with appropriate labelling requirements?

- What products are on display which are clearly labelled as not suitable for feeding young infants (e.g. powdered, evaporated or sweetened condensed milks)?

- Note any unsuitable products which might be used for feeding young infants displayed with, or in the immediate vicinity of, infant formula (e.g. powdered/skim milks).

- Note any coupons, special prices, discount offers, etc.

- Note any in-store promotion for infant feeding products.

Reference

1. *Protecting, promoting and support breast-feeding: the special role of maternity services.* A joint WHO/UNICEF statement, op. cit.

Sample questionnaires

Annex 8

1. Sample questionnaire for the competent national authorities
    (government leaders in health, social welfare and related sectors) 77

2. Sample questionnaire for professional associations,
    nongovernmental organizations, and consumer
    and mother-support groups 85

3. Sample questionnaire for mothers in hospital maternity wards 93

4. Sample questionnaire for directors of nursing, medical directors,
    and administrators in hospitals, wards and clinics 99

5. Sample questionnaire for health facility purchasing officers 107

6. Sample questionnaire for health professionals working in
    maternity hospitals, wards and clinics 111

7. Sample questionnaire for community-based health professionals 119

8. Sample questionnaire for retailers and retail pharmacists 127

N.B. For all questionnaires, additional space may be required to answer completely all
the points covered.

Sample questionnaires

1 Sample questionnaire for the competent national authorities (government leaders in health, social welfare and related sectors)

Please include copies of documents where available.

1. What national and local measures have been taken to give effect to the International Code of Marketing of Breast-milk Substitutes?

2. What impact have these measures had in health care facilities and communities on:
   (a) The marketing of breast-milk substitutes?
   (b) Advertising or promotion of breast-milk substitutes to the general public?
   (c) The protection and promotion of breast-feeding?
   (d) The appropriate preparation and use of breast-milk substitutes?

   _____

3. Are there any products covered within the scope of the International Code which have been **omitted** from national measures?

   Yes   ☐ *No*   ☐ *Don't know* ☐ *If yes*, please explain.

   _____

4. Are there any products Not covered within the scope of the International Code which have been **included** in national measures?

   Yes   ☐ *No*   ☐ *Don't know* ☐ *If yes*, please explain.

   _____

5. **Regarding the provision of samples and gifts by manufacturers and distributors to pregnant and lactating women:**

    (a) What impact have the national measures had on the provision of samples and gifts?

    _____

    (b) Describe any factors which you feel have **facilitated** or **hindered** implementation of the national measures in the area of samples and gifts.

    _____

6. **Regarding information on infant feeding given to pregnant women and families:**

    (a) Do the competent authorities take responsibility for ensuring objective and consistent information on infant feeding which is given to pregnant women and families?

    Yes   ☐   _No_   ☐

    (b) _If yes_, who takes this responsibility and how is it carried out?

    _____

    (c) _If no_, what alternative arrangement is made to ensure that information is objective and consistent?

    _____

    (d) Through what mechanisms do the competent authorities review or exert control over the content and dissemination of materials for pregnant women and families which are produced by others, including manufacturers of products within the scope of the Code?

    _____

    (e) Are there any donations or distribution of educational materials by manufacturers for use by pregnant women or families? _If yes_, under what conditions?

    _____

7. **Regarding information about breast-feeding and infant nutrition that is used for the education of health workers:**

(a) Do the competent authorities take responsibility for information about breast-feeding and infant nutrition that is included in education for health workers?

Yes ☐ Answer 7(b) - (d) *No* ☐ Go to 7(e)

(b) *If yes*, describe how the responsibility is carried out.

_____

(c) What educational materials (e.g. pamphlets, books, videos, audio cassettes, in-service courses) on breast-feeding do the competent authorities produce for health workers?

_____

(d) For which health workers are educational materials prepared?

_____

(e) Who else contributes to materials about breast-feeding and infant nutrition that is included in education for health providers?

_____

(f) Do national measures prohibit or permit the participation of infant food manufacturers (e.g. giving lectures) in educating health professionals?

_____

(g) Describe the impact national measures have had on manufacturers' involvement in health worker education, if permitted, and the factors which have **facilitated** and **hindered** implementation of national measures in this regard.

_____

(h)   If donations of educational equipment or materials have been made by manufacturers, do they bear images or information about products in addition to the company's logo?

If yes, give examples.

_____

(i)   Are educational materials required to include the information specified in the Code's Article 4.2?

_____

8.   **Regarding the display and promotion of breast-milk substitutes in health facilities:**

(a)   How have the display and promotion of breast-milk substitutes in health facilities been addressed by the competent authorities?

_____

(b)   What has been the impact of the action taken?

_____

(c)   What factors have **facilitated** or **hindered** implementation of national measures in this area?

_____

(d)   Is feeding with infant formula demonstrated only by health workers and limited only to mothers or family members who need to use it?

_____

9. **Regarding donation of supplies of breast-milk substitutes and equipment to health facilities:**

    (a) Are donations of supplies of breast-milk substitutes and equipment made by manufacturers or distributors to health care facilities? Are these donations monitored by the competent authorities?

    _____

    (b) *If yes*, describe the quantities and donors and the mechanism by which monitoring occurs.

    _____

    (c) Describe the impact monitoring has had on donations of breast-milk substitutes and equipment to health facilities.

    _____

    (d) Describe the factors which have **facilitated** or **hindered** action in this area.

    _____

10. **Regarding the promotion of breast-feeding:**

    (a) How do the competent authorities define their role in promoting breast-feeding and what measures are they taking for this purpose?

    _____

    (b) Have national measures to implement the International Code changed the way breast-feeding is promoted?

    _____

11. **Regarding monitoring of national measures:**

    (a) Do the competent authorities monitor implementation of national measures to give effect to the International Code?

    Yes ☐ Answer 11(b) - (f)   *No* ☐   Go to 11 (d)

(b)   *If yes*, what action is taken to deal with breaches of national measures and to what authority should alleged breaches be reported?

_____

(c)   As part of monitoring national measures, are the competent authorities directly or indirectly in contact with any of the following:

Manufacturers   *Yes*   □ *No*   □ *Don't know*   □

Professional groups   *Yes*   □ *No*   □ *Don't know*   □

Consumer organisations   *Yes*   □ *No*   □ *Don't know*   □

(d)   Have any individuals or agencies ever reported alleged breaches?

_____

(e)   *If yes*, attach details of the number and nature of the reports.

_____

(f)   What action was taken when alleged breaches were reported?

_____

12.   **Finally, please consider the overall effectiveness of the national and local measures that have been taken to give effect to the International Code:**

(a)   In your opinion, how effective have the measures been in fulfilling the aim of the International Code (Article 1)? Please explain you answer.

_____

(b) Have any factors **facilitated** or **hindered** the implementation of these measures at a local or national level?

Yes ☐ *No* ☐ *Don't know* ☐

If yes, please list each factor and explain how it has facilitated or hindered implementation.

_____

(c) Are there any aspects of national measures which you feel have the potential to cause harm to infants? *If yes*, please describe.

_____

(d) Please record any additional comments you have concerning the implementation of the International Code in your country.

_____

OBSERVATIONS/SUMMARY RESULTS.

OBSERVATIONS/SUMMARY RESULTS *cont.*

2 Sample questionnaire for professional associations, nongovernmental organizations, and consumer and mother-support groups

1. Is the aim of the International Code reflected in national health **policy**?

    Yes ☐   *No* ☐   *Don't know* ☐ Please explain your answer.

    _____

2. Is the aim of the International Code reflected in national health **practice**?

    Yes ☐   *No* ☐   *Don't know* ☐ Please explain your answer.

    _____

3. Are there any aspects of the International Code which have been omitted from national measures?

    Yes ☐   *No* ☐   *Don't know* ☐ *If yes*, please explain.

    _____

4. What impact have the national measures to implement the International Code had on:

    (a)   The marketing of breast-milk substitutes?

    _____

    (b)   Protection of breast-feeding?

    _____

(c)   Promotion of breast-feeding?

_____

(d)   Appropriate preparation and use of breast-milk substitutes?

_____

(e)   The advertising or promotion of products within the scope of the International Code to the general public in print media, radio, television, handouts to pregnant women and new mothers, etc.?

_____

(f)   The provision and content of information, to health professionals, about products within the scope of the Code?

_____

(g)   The provision and content of information provided to pregnant women and mothers?

_____

Regarding the provision of samples and gifts to pregnant women and parents of young children:

5.   What impact have national measures had on the provision of samples, i.e. single or small quantities of products within the scope of the Code provided without cost to pregnant women, mothers or their families?

_____

6. Describe the factors which have **facilitated** or **hindered** implementation of the national measures regarding samples.

_____

7. What impact have national measures had on the provision of gifts by companies to mothers?

_____

8. Describe the factors which have **facilitated** or **hindered** implementation of national measures regarding gifts.

_____

Regarding the marketing of products within the scope of national measures:

9. What impact have the national measures had on the **marketing** of products within their scope to the general public?

_____

10. Describe the factors which have **facilitated** or **hindered** implementation of national measures regarding marketing of products within the scope of the Code.

_____

11. Are you aware of any instances in the area of **marketing** in which manufacturers appear to have breached national measures?

    Yes ☐   _No_ ☐

    If yes, please describe these instances and, if possible, attach copies of relevant reports.

_____

Regarding the display and promotion in health facilities of products within the scope of the International Code:

12.   What impact have the national measures had on the display and promotion of products in maternal and child health facilities?

_____

13.   Describe the factors which have **facilitated** or **hindered** implementation of national measures in this area.

_____

Regarding product donations to maternal and child health facilities:

14.   What impact have national measures had on the donation of products within the scope of the Code?

_____

15.   What factors have **facilitated** or **hindered** the implementation of the national measures in this area?

_____

Regarding the protection and support of breast-feeding:

16.   How effective have national measures been in promoting and protecting breast-feeding?
       Very effective   ☐   _Effective_   ☐   _Not very effective_   ☐

_____

17. What factors have **facilitated** or **hindered** implementation of national measures to protect and promote breast-feeding?

_____

18. Are your members made aware of national measures to give effect to the International Code?

Yes ☐ *No* ☐ *Don't know* ☐

If yes, please describe the procedures by which you make your employees/members aware of national measures.

_____

Regarding monitoring of implementation of the International Code:

19. Is adherence to national measures being monitored in your country?

Yes ☐ *No* (go to 31) ☐ *Don't know* (go to 31) ☐

If yes, who is monitoring adherence and how effective is this monitoring?

_____

20. Have you ever informed the competent authorities of any activities which you considered to be incompatible with national measures, e.g. display of products within the scope of national measures in facilities of the health care system, financial or material inducements to health workers to promote products?

Yes ☐ *No* ☐

If yes, please give details and describe what action was taken as a result of your report?

_____

Regarding the overall effectiveness of the implementation and monitoring of national measures adopted to give effect to the International Code:

21.   In your opinion, how effective have the national measures been?

_____

22.   Are there any aspects of the national measures which you feel have the potential to cause harm to infants? *If yes*, please describe.

_____

23.   Are there any relevant aspects or issues which you feel should be addressed by the national measures and are not? *If yes*, please describe.

_____

24.   Please record any additional comments you have concerning implementation of the International Code in your country.

_____

OBSERVATIONS/ASSESSMENT RESULTS

OBSERVATIONS/ASSESSMENT RESULTS *cont.*

3 Sample questionnaire for mothers in hospital maternity wards

1. What has your baby been fed in the past 24 hours?

   ☐ Breast milk only?

   ☐ Mostly breast milk, but baby has had some infant formula, glucose and/or plain water?

   ☐ Infant formula (including specialised formula) only?

   ☐ Mostly infant formula, but baby has had some breast milk?

   _____

2. Is the answer to question 1 the same as how your baby has been fed since birth?

   Yes ☐ *No* ☐

   If no, can you briefly explain why there has been a change?

   _____

3. If your baby has been kept in a nursery at any time, what did the staff do when the baby was hungry?

   ☐ They brought baby to me to feed.

   ☐ They let me know and I went to the nursery to feed.

   ☐ They gave baby infant formula.

   ☐ They gave baby my expressed breast milk.

   ☐ They gave baby glucose water.

   ☐ They gave baby plain water.

   ☐ I don't know.

   _____

4.   If your baby has been fed by the staff, were you informed before this happened?

☐   *Yes*, I was informed.

☐   *Yes*, I signed a consent form.

☐   *No*, I was not asked.

☐   I don't know.

5.   Has any member of the staff encouraged you to breast-feed and counselled you in this regard?

Yes   ☐   *No*   ☐

If yes, who? (doctor, nurse, etc).

6.   Since you have been in the maternity unit, have any of the following items been made available to you by the hospital? (Check all that are relevant to you).

☐   Pamphlets/booklets on breast-feeding your baby.

☐   Pamphlets/booklets on bottle-feeding your baby.

☐   Pamphlets/booklets on caring for your baby.

☐   Video/audiotape (either to watch or copy to keep) on breast-feeding your baby.

☐   Video/audiotape (either to watch or copy to keep) on bottle-feeding your baby.

☐   Video/audiotape (either to watch or copy to keep) on caring for your baby.

7.   Did any of these materials mention, show pictures or advertise any product name of an infant formula, feeding bottle or teat (nipple)? Please tick, and if possible write name of product/s.

☐   Pamphlets/booklets on breast-feeding.

☐   Pamphlets/booklets on bottle-feeding.

☐   Pamphlets/booklets on caring for baby.

☐ Video on breast-feeding.

☐ Video on bottle-feeding.

☐ Video on caring for baby.

---

8. For the first few weeks after you go home from hospital, how do you plan to feed your baby?

☐ Exclusive breast-feeding.

☐ Mostly breast-feeding, some formula.

☐ Mostly formula feeding, some breast milk.

☐ Completely formula feeding.

---

9. If you plan to feed your baby infant formula, has any member of the hospital staff talked to you (or shown you) how to prepare infant formula?

Yes ☐   *No* ☐

If yes, was there an explanation of the potential health hazards?

---

10. Have you ever been offered a sample of infant formula or has it ever been suggested that you should reduce your breast-feeding? By whom? For what reason?

---

11. Have you ever been told your baby "needed" formula? *If yes*, by whom? Why? Were you given free formula? What quantity?

---

12.   Is formula ever better for your baby? When? Why? Who told you so?

OBSERVATIONS/ASSESSMENT RESULTS

OBSERVATIONS/ASSESSMENT RESULTS *cont.*

4 Sample questionnaire for directors of nursing, medical directors, and administrators in maternity hospitals, wards and clinics

1. How many maternity beds does your health facility have and how many births are there per year?

   _____

2. Does your facility have a written breast-feeding policy that is routinely communicated to all health care staff?

   _____

3. What is the average length of stay:
   - For normal deliveries?
   - For Caesarean deliveries?
   - For premature babies?
   - For mothers of premature babies?

   _____

4. What percentage of women in your facility initiate breast-feeding?

   _____

5.   What percentage of women are exclusively [1] or predominantly [2] breast-feeding on discharge from your facility?

_____

6.   During their stay in the health care facility, what percentage of breast-fed babies get at least one complementary feed of:

   • Water?

   • Glucose water?

   • Infant formula?

_____

7.   Are you aware of the International Code of Marketing of Breast-milk Substitutes?

_____

8.   What national and local measures have been taken to give effect to the International Code?

_____

9.   What impact have these measures had on:

   • The general marketing of breast-milk substitutes, bottles and teats?

   • The protection and promotion of breast-feeding?

   • The appropriate preparation and use of breast-milk substitutes?

_____

_____

[1] Exclusive breast-feeding means that infants receive breast milk (including milk expressed or from a wet-nurse); it allows infants to receive drops, syrups (vitamins, minerals, medicines); it does not allow infants to receive anything else.

[2] Predominant breast-feeding means that infants receive breast milk (including milk expressed or from a wet-nurse) as their predominant source of nourishment; it allows infants to receive liquids (water, water-based drinks, fruit juice, oral rehydration salts), ritual fluids and drops or syrups (vitamins, minerals, medicines); it does not allow the infant to receive anything else (in particular, non-human milk, and food-based fluids).

Regarding the display and promotion in health facilities of products within the scope of the International Code:

10.   Does your facility have a policy on the display and promotion to mothers of breast-milk substitutes, bottles or teats, directly or indirectly, through company posters, materials, free offers, etc.?

   Yes ☐   *No* ☐   *If yes*, please describe.

   _____

11.   *If yes*, what impact has this policy had on breast-feeding promotion in your facility?

   _____

12.   What factors have **facilitated** or **hindered** having and implementing such a policy?

   _____

Regarding information on infant feeding which is given to pregnant women and families:

13.   Does your facility have a policy regarding donations by manufacturers and distributors of educational materials covered by the Code?

   Yes ☐   *No* ☐   *If yes*, please describe.

   _____

14.   *If yes*, what impact has this policy had?

   _____

15.   If donations of materials are made, do they bear product names or information about any products manufactured by the company which donated them?

   _____

16.   What factors have **facilitated** or **hindered** having and implementing such a policy?

_____

Regarding the provision of samples and gifts by manufacturers and distributors to pregnant and lactating women:

17.   Does your facility have a policy concerning the provision of samples or gifts to pregnant women or new mothers (e.g. infant formula, feeding bottles, teats, baby items or toys bearing company logo)?

         Yes ☐   *No* ☐   Please describe.

_____

18.   *If yes*, what impact has this policy had?

_____

19.   What factors have facilitated or hindered having and implementing such a policy?

         Who is responsible for monitoring compliance with the policy?

_____

Regarding company personnel and mothers:

20.   Do personnel from manufacturers of products within the scope of the Code have any contact with mothers at your facility, or are any health care personnel provided or paid for by manufacturers.

_____

Regarding the procurement of breast-milk substitutes and infant feeding equipment ("products") by health facilities:

21. How is the facility and its staff informed by the manufacturers of new or existing products?

_____

22. Who decides which products will be used in the facility?

_____

23. How is this decision made?

_____

24. How often is the decision reviewed?

_____

25. What products are currently used?

_____

26. How are the products used by this facility usually obtained?

_____

27. On average, how much is paid for each can, sachet and/or bottle of ready-to-feed infant formula?

_____

28.   Does the facility receive some or all of its infant formula, feeding bottles or teats through donations or at a subsidised price?

Yes ☐ *No* ☐ *Don't know* ☐

29.   *If yes,*

- What quantity of donated or subsidised formula does the facility receive per month?
- In what form(s) do the donated supplies come, e.g. ready-to-feed, tins of powder?
- Is there an order form / receipt / invoice?
- Are the donations monitored? By whom?

Regarding funding by manufacturers or distributors of products within the scope of the Code of research, fellowships, study tours, conferences, etc.:

30.   Does the facility or any member of its staff receive funding from manufacturers or distributors to conduct research in any aspect of infant health?

Yes   ☐ *No*   ☐ *Don't know* ☐

If yes, please give details

---

31.   Have manufacturers or distributors ever supported any of the following:

Fellowships	*Yes* ☐ *No* ☐ *Don't know* ☐
Study tours	*Yes* ☐ *No* ☐ *Don't know* ☐
Conference attendance	*Yes* ☐ *No* ☐ *Don't know* ☐
In-service seminars	*Yes* ☐ *No* ☐ *Don't know* ☐

If yes to any of the above, please give details

---

32.   Are funding recipients required to disclose contributions to their institutions?

Yes   ☐   *No*   ☐ *Don't know* ☐

---

33.   Are manufacturers and distributors required to disclose to institutions the funding they provide to staff?

Yes ☐   *No* ☐ *Don't know* ☐

Regarding manufacturers' compliance with national measures:

34.   Are you aware of any instances in the area of marketing in which manufacturers' practices appear to have been at variance with national measures to give effect to the International Code?

Yes ☐ *No* ☐ *If yes*, please describe these instances.

Regarding the overall effectiveness of the implementation
and monitoring of national measures:

35.   In your opinion, how effective have national measures been in fulfilling the aim of the International Code (Article 1)?

36.   Are there any aspects of national measures which you feel have the potential to cause harm to infants? *If yes*, please describe.

37.   Are there any relevant aspects or issues which you feel should be addressed by national measures and are not? *If yes*, please describe.

OBSERVATIONS/ASSESSMENT RESULTS

5 Sample questionnaire for health facility purchasing officers

Regarding the procurement of breast-milk substitutes and infant feeding equipment ("products") by your facility:

1.   How is the facility and its staff informed by manufacturers of new or existing products?

_____

2.   Who decides which products will be used in the facility?

_____

3.   How is this decision made?

_____

4.   How often is the decision reviewed?

_____

5.   What products are currently used?

_____

6.   How are the products used by the facility normally obtained?

_____

7.   On average, how much is paid for each can, sachet and/or bottle of ready-to-feed infant formula?

_____

8.   Does the facility receive some or all of its infant formula or other products within the scope of the Code through donations or at a subsidised price?

      Yes   ☐   *No*   ☐

9.   *If yes,*

      (a)   What quantity of donated or subsidised formula does the facility receive per month?

_____

      (b)   In what form(s) do the donated supplies come, e.g. ready-to-feed, tins of powder?

_____

      (c)   Is there an order form / receipt / invoice?

_____

      (d)   Are donations monitored and by whom?

_____

Regarding manufacturers' compliance with national measures:

10.   Are you aware of any instances in the area of marketing in which manufacturers' practices appear to have been at variance with national action to give effect to the International Code of Marketing of Breast-milk Substitutes?

      Yes   ☐   *No*   ☐   *If yes,* please describe these instances.

_____

OBSERVATIONS/ASSESSMENT RESULTS

OBSERVATIONS/ASSESSMENT RESULTS *cont.*

6 Sample questionnaire for health professionals working in maternity hospitals, wards and clinics

This sample questionnaire can be used to interview health professionals (e.g. medical staff and specialists, midwives, nurses, etc.) in the health care facilities visited during the review process. It could also be mailed to all health care facilities with at least 500 births per year.

POSTAL CODE/REGION _____

1.　　Are you aware of the International Code of Marketing of Breast-milk Substitutes?

　　　Yes　☐　　*No*　☐

2.　　Are you familiar with the content of the national and local measures that have been adopted to give effect to the International Code of Marketing of Breast-milk Substitutes?

　　　Yes　☐　　*No*　☐

3.　　Was there any formal procedure at your facility by which you were made familiar with these measures as they relate to health workers' responsibilities?

　　　Yes　☐　　*No*　☐

4.　　Is there a copy of these measures readily available at your facility for you to read?

　　　Yes　☐　　*No*　☐

5.　　In your opinion, what impact have these measures had at your facility on:

　　　(a)　　The protection and promotion of breast-feeding?

　　　_____

　　　(b)　　Promotion of breast-milk substitutes, feeding bottles and teats?

　　　_____

(c)   The appropriate preparation and use of breast-milk substitutes?

Regarding the display and promotion of breast-milk substitutes in health facilities:

6.   Does your facility have any displays, posters, or materials which promote breast-milk substitutes, bottles or teats to the mothers in your care?

Yes   ☐   *No*   ☐   *If yes*, please describe.

Regarding information on infant feeding which is given to pregnant women and families:

7.   Does your facility accept donations of parenting and/or infant feeding educational materials which are produced or sponsored by manufacturers of products within the scope of the Code?

Yes   ☐   *No*   ☐   *Don't know* ☐

(a)   *If yes*, do any materials bear product names, or information about any products manufactured by the company which donated, produced or sponsored them?

Yes   ☐ *No*   ☐   *If yes*, please describe.

(b)   *If yes*, is the content monitored / approved before distribution?

Please give details.

Regarding free or subsidised provision of supplies of infant formula or other products within the scope of the Code:

8.   Is any infant formula or other product within the scope of the Code given to the facility free or at subsidised cost?

Yes   ☐   *No*   ☐   *Don't know* ☐

If yes, give details.

Regarding samples and gifts to mothers:

9.   When mothers are leaving your facility, do they receive samples of infant formula or other products within the scope of the Code?

Yes   ☐   *No*   ☐   *Don't know* ☐

If yes,

(a)   Which mothers are given samples?

_____

(b)   Under what circumstances are breast-feeding mothers specifically given samples?

_____

10.   When mothers are leaving your facility, do they receive discharge packs which contain any discount or special offers for samples of formula or other products within the scope of the Code?

Yes   ☐   *No*   ☐   *Don't know* ☐

If yes, please give details.

_____

11.   Do any mothers at your facility receive gifts (e.g. toys, baby items or equipment) which are donated, produced or sponsored by manufacturers?

Yes   ☐   *No*   ☐

If yes, do these gifts bear any product or company identification, e.g. name or logo? Please describe.

_____

Regarding manufacturers personnel and mothers:

12.   Do personnel from manufacturers of products within the scope of the Code have any contact with mothers at the facility?

_____

Regarding samples and gifts to health workers:

13.   Do manufacturers and distributors of products within the scope of the Code give health workers product samples or gifts?

    (a)   Have you encountered this?   *Yes* ☐   *No* ☐

    (b)   If you experienced this personally, how did you respond?

_____

Regarding funding of research, fellowships, study tours, conferences, etc.:

14.   Have manufacturers or distributors ever offered you or supported your participation in any of the following?

Fellowships	*Yes*	☐	*No*	☐
Study tours	*Yes*	☐	*No*	☐
Conference attendance	*Yes*	☐	*No*	☐
In-service seminars	*Yes*	☐	*No*	☐

_____

15.   *If yes* to any of the above, please give details

_____

16.   Are you required to disclose such funding to your health care facility?

       Yes   ☐   *No*   ☐   *Don't know* ☐

_____

17.   Are manufacturers and distributors also required to disclose such funding?

       Yes   ☐   *No*   ☐   *Don't know* ☐

_____

Regarding manufacturers' compliance with national measures:

18.   Are you aware of any instances in the area of marketing where manufacturers' practices appear to have been at variance with national action taken to give effect to the International Code?

       Yes   ☐   *No*   ☐   *If yes*, please describe these instances.

_____

Regarding the overall effectiveness of implementation and monitoring of national measures to give effect to the International Code:

19.   In your opinion, how effective have national measures been in fulfilling the aim of the Code (Article 1)?

_____

20.   Are there any aspects of national measures which you feel have the potential to cause harm to infants? *If yes*, please describe.

_____

21.   Are there any aspects or issues which you feel should be addressed by national measures and are not? *If yes*, please describe.

OBSERVATIONS/ASSESSMENT RESULTS

OBSERVATIONS/ASSESSMENT RESULTS *cont.*

7 Sample questionnaire for community-based health professionals

This questionnaire can be used to interview personnel in centres visited during the review process. It can also be mailed to all centres with at least 500 births per year.

POSTAL CODE/REGION _____

1.   Are you aware of the International Code of Marketing of Breast-milk Substitutes?

       Yes   ☐   *No*   ☐

2.   Are you familiar with the content of national and local measures that have been adopted to give effect to the International Code of Marketing of Breast-milk Substitutes?

       Yes   ☐   *No*   ☐   *Don't know*   ☐

3.   Was there any formal procedure by which you became familiar with these measures as they relate to health workers' responsibilities?

       Yes   ☐   *No*   ☐

4.   Has your professional association adopted a formal policy on the International Code or the national measures taken to give effect to it?

       Yes   ☐   *No*   ☐   *Don't know*   ☐

       I am not a member of a professional association ☐

5.   Is there a copy of these measures readily available for you to read?

       Yes   ☐   *No*   ☐   *Don't know*   ☐

6.   In your opinion, what impact have these measures had on:

(a)   The protection and promotion of breast-feeding?

_____

(b)   The marketing and promotion of breast-milk substitutes, feeding bottles and teats?

_____

(c)   The appropriate preparation and use of breast-milk substitutes?

_____

Regarding the display and promotion of breast-milk substitutes in health facilities:

7.   Does your facility have any displays, posters, or materials which promote breast-milk substitutes, bottles or teats to the mothers in its care?

Yes   ☐   *No*   ☐   *Please describe.*

_____

Regarding information on infant feeding which is given to pregnant women and families:

8.   Do you or your facility accept donations of educational materials dealing with the feeding of infants which are produced or sponsored by manufacturers and distributors and intended for pregnant women and mothers of infants and young children?

Yes   ☐   *No*   ☐   *Don't know*   ☐

(a)   *If yes*, do any materials bear product names, or information about any products of the manufacturers which donated, produced or sponsored the materials?

Yes   ☐   *No*   ☐   Please describe.

(b)   *If yes*, is the content of the materials monitored / approved before distribution? Please give details.

(c)   Do you or your facility require that the materials contain clear information on all the points specified in the Code's Article 4.2?

Regarding free or subsidised provision of infant formula or other products within the scope of the Code:

9.   Is any infant formula or other product within the scope of the Code given to you or your facility free or at subsidised cost?

Yes   ☐   *No*   ☐   *Don't know*   ☐

If yes, give details.

Regarding samples and gifts to mothers:

10.   Do you or your facility ever give parents samples of infant formula or other products within the scope of the Code?

Yes   ☐   *No*   ☐   *Don't know*   ☐

If yes,

(a)   Which mothers are given the samples?

_____

(b)   Under what circumstances are breast-feeding mothers given samples?

_____

11.   Do you or your facility ever give parents discharge packs containing any discount or special offers for samples of infant formula and/or feeding equipment?

Yes   ☐   *No*   ☐   *Don't know*   ☐

If yes, please give details.

_____

12.   Do mothers at your facility receive toys, baby items or equipment which are donated, produced or sponsored by manufacturers?

Yes   ☐   *No*   ☐

If yes, do these gifts bear any product or company identification, e.g. name or logo? *Please describe.*

_____

Regarding manufacturers' personnel and mothers:

13.   Do representatives of manufacturers of products within the scope of the Code have any contact with mothers?

_____

Regarding samples and gifts to health workers:

14.   Do manufacturers marketing products within the scope of the Code give health workers samples or gifts?

    (a)   Have you encountered this?   *Yes* ☐   *No* ☐

    (b)   If you experienced this personally, how did you respond?

Regarding funding of research, fellowships, study tours, conferences, etc.:

15.   Have manufacturers or distributors ever offered you or supported your participation in any of the following:

Fellowships	*Yes* ☐	*No* ☐	*Don't know* ☐
Study tours	*Yes* ☐	*No* ☐	*Don't know* ☐
Conference attendance	*Yes* ☐	*No* ☐	*Don't know* ☐
In-service seminars	*Yes* ☐	*No* ☐	*Don't know* ☐

16   *If yes* to any of the above, please give details.

17.   Are you required to disclose such funding to your employer?

    Yes ☐   *No* ☐   *Don't know* ☐

18.   Are manufacturers and distributors required to disclose such support?

       Yes   ☐   *No*   ☐   *Don't know*   ☐

Regarding manufacturers' compliance with national measures:

19.   Are you aware of any instances in the area of marketing where manufacturers' practices appear to have been at variance with national action taken to give effect to the International Code?

       Yes   ☐   *No*   ☐   *If yes*, please describe these instances.

Regarding the overall effectiveness of the implementation and monitoring of the national measures to give effect to the International Code:

20.   In your opinion, how effective have measures been in fulfilling the aim of the International Code (Article 1)?

---

21.   Are there any aspects of national measures which you feel have the potential to cause harm to infants? *If yes*, please give details.

---

22.   Are there any relevant aspects or issues which you feel should be addressed by national measures and are not? *If yes*, please describe.

OBSERVATIONS/ASSESSMENT RESULTS

OBSERVATIONS/ASSESSMENT RESULTS *cont.*

8 Sample questionnaire for retailers and retail pharmacists

Postal code _____

1. Are you aware of the International Code of Marketing of Breast-milk Substitutes?

   Yes ☐ *No* ☐

2. Are you familiar with the content of the national and local measures that have been adopted to give effect to the International Code of Marketing of Breast-milk Substitutes?

   Yes ☐ *No* ☐ *Don't know* ☐

3. Was there any formal procedure by which you became familiar with these measures as they relate to retailers' responsibilities?

   Yes ☐ *No* ☐

4. Is there a copy of these measures readily available for you to read?

   Yes ☐ *No* ☐ *Don't know* ☐

5. Do these measures specify any specific responsibilities for retailers?

   Yes ☐ *No* ☐ *Don't know* ☐

   If yes, What are these responsibilities?

   _____

6. Do you ensure that your practices are in accordance with national measures?

   Yes ☐ *No* ☐ *If yes*, how do you monitor your practices?

   _____

7.   Does your association (or company/buying group) have a policy with regard to the International Code or national measures taken to give effect to it?

    Yes   ☐   *No*   ☐   *Don't know*   ☐

Regarding advertising and promotion:

8.   Is the manner in which you sell infant formula and other products within the scope of the Code any different from the way you sell other products?

    Yes   ☐   *No*   ☐

    If yes

    (a)   How does the sale of infant formula and other products within the scope of the Code differ?

    _____

    (b)   Is there any attempt to draw attention to products within the scope of the Code by displaying them prominently or including promotional messages in the immediate vicinity?

        Yes ☐   *No* ☐

    _____

    (c)   Is infant formula easily differentiated from other products intended for feeding older infants and young children?

        Yes ☐   *No* ☐

    _____

9.   Is the manner in which you advertise, promote and sell infant feeding equipment (e.g. bottles and teats) any different from the way other products are advertised and sold.

    Yes   ☐   *No*   ☐

If yes,

(a)   How does the sale of infant feeding equipment differ?

_____

(b)   Who decided that it should be different?

_____

10.   How often would infant formula and other products within the scope of the Code be sold at a special price in this store?

_____

11.   Do you promote infant formula and other products within the scope of the Code through the media?
Yes ☐ *No* ☐

12.   Are there any quotas for the sale of infant formula?
Yes ☐ *No* ☐

13.   Are there any quotas for the sale of any manufacturer's feeding bottles and/or teats?
Yes ☐ *No* ☐

14.   Are there bonuses, or any other sales incentives, for the sale of products within the scope of the Code?
Yes ☐ *No* ☐

15.   Are there **bonuses**, or any other sales incentives, for the sale of any manufacturer's feeding bottles and/or teats?
Yes ☐ *No* ☐

16. Do manufacturers or distributors of infant formula provide information on restrictions as to how their products should be marketed?

    Yes ☐ *No* ☐ *If yes*, please describe:

    _____

17. Do manufacturers or distributors of feeding bottles and teats provide information on restrictions as to how their products should be marketed?

    Yes ☐ *No* ☐ *If yes*, please describe:

    _____

18. Are infant formula and other products within the scope of the Code displayed for sale together with other products, e.g. herbal teas, starchy gruels, sweetened condensed milk, and follow-up formula, thereby possibly contributing to these products being incorrectly perceived as appropriate breast-milk substitutes?

    Yes ☐ *No* ☐

    _____

Regarding information on infant feeding which is given to pregnant women and families:

19. Do you or your retail outlet distribute infant feeding and/or parenting educational materials which are produced or sponsored by infant food manufacturers?

    Yes ☐ No ☐ *Don't know* ☐

    (a) *If yes*, do any materials bear product names, or information about any products produced by the company which donated, produced or sponsored them?

         Yes ☐ *No* ☐ *If yes*, please describe.

    _____

(b)   *If yes*, is the content monitored/approved by the competent authority before distribution? Please give details.

Regarding free or subsidised provision of infant formula or other products within the scope of the Code:

20.   Is any infant formula or any other product within the scope of the Code given to you or your retail outlet free or at subsidised cost?

Yes   ☐   *No*   ☐   *Don't know* ☐   *If yes*, give details.

Regarding samples and gifts to mothers:

21.   Do you or your retail outlet ever give parents samples of infant formula and/or feeding equipment?

Yes   ☐   *No*   ☐   *Don't know* ☐   *If yes*,

(a)   Which mothers are given the samples?

(b)   Under what circumstances are breast-feeding mothers given samples?

22.   Does your retail outlet ever offer discount or special offers for samples of formula and/or feeding equipment?

Yes   ☐   *No*   ☐   *Don't know* ☐   *If yes*, please give details.

23. Does your retail outlet ever give to pregnant women or parents toys, baby items or equipment which have been donated, produced or sponsored by infant food manufacturers?

Yes ☐   *No* ☐

If yes, do these gifts bear any product or company identification, e.g. name or logo?

Please describe.

Regarding manufacturers' personnel and mothers:

24. Do personnel from manufacturers of products within the scope of the Code have any contact with mothers at the retail outlet?

Regarding manufacturers' compliance with national measures:

25. Are you aware of any instances in the area of marketing where manufacturers' practices appear to have been at variance with national action taken to give effect to the International Code of Marketing of Breast-milk Substitutes?

Yes ☐   *No* ☐   *If yes*, please describe these instances.

---

26. Have you ever informed the competent authority of any activities which you thought were incompatible with national measures?

Yes ☐   *No* ☐   *If yes*,

(a)   Please give details.

(b)   What action was taken as a result?

Regarding the overall effectiveness of implementation and monitoring of national measures adopted to give effect to the International Code:

27.   In your opinion, how effective have national measures been?

---

28.   Are there any aspects of national measures which you feel have the potential to cause harm to infants? *If yes*, please outline.

---

29.   Are there any relevant aspects or issues which you feel should be addressed by national measures and are not? *If yes*, please describe.

OBSERVATIONS/ASSESSMENT RESULTS

OBSERVATIONS/ASSESSMENT RESULTS *cont.*

www.ingramcontent.com/pod-product-compliance
Lightning Source LLC
Chambersburg PA
CBHW061105210326
41597CB00021B/3980